Emergency Department Handbook

Children and adolescents with mental health problems

Emergency Department Handbook

Children and adolescents with mental health problems

Edited by Tony Kaplan

RCPsych Publications

© The Royal College of Psychiatrists 2009

RCPsych Publications is an imprint of the Royal College of Psychiatrists,
17 Belgrave Square, London SW1X 8PG
http://www.rcpsych.ac.uk

British Library Cataloguing-in-Publication Data.
A catalogue record for this book is available from the British Library.
ISBN 978 1 901671 73 2

Distributed in North America by Publishers Storage and Shipping Company.

Printed by Bell & Bain Limited, Glasgow, UK.

Contents

Acknowledgements

This book is derived from the work of an inter-collegiate group that met under the auspices of the Child and Adolescent Faculty Executive of the Royal College of Psychiatrists, chaired by Dr Tony Kaplan, to examine the delivery of child and adolescent mental health services in the setting of emergency departments in the UK. We took reference from existing Royal College of Psychiatrists' Council Reports CR64, CR118 and CR122. This culminated in the Faculty document *Child and Adolescent Mental Health Problems in the Emergency Department and the Services to Deal with These* (Royal College of Psychiatrists, 2006a). Members of the Working Group were: Josie Brown, Lois Colling, Tony Kaplan, Catherine Lavelle, Helen Stuart and Julie Waine (all Royal College of Psychiatrists, Child and Adolescent Faculty); Ian Maconochie and Avril Washington (Royal College of Paediatrics and Child Health); and Diana Hulbert (College of Emergency Medicine/British Association of Emergency Medicine).

I am very grateful to Dr Tricia Brennan for the trouble she took in proof-reading the final draft of this book, Dr Sebastian Kraemer for his enduring commitment, Dr Peter Bruggen for being the inspiration behind Chapter 3, and Drs Susannah Fairweather and Quentin Spender for their astute editorial comments.

Special thanks

The chapter authors are especially grateful for contributions from the following: Chapter 2, Tony Kaplan for the subsection on the importance of attachment; Chapter 4, Lois Colling for the subsection on anxiety, Diana Hulbert for the subsection on altered consciousness/altered mental status, Tony Kaplan for the subsections on acute stress reactions and post-traumatic stress disorder, and psychosis, and Catherine Lavelle for the subsections on the side-effects of psychotropic medication and factors increasing index of concern in substance misuse; Chapter 5, Quentin Spender for the Differential Grid for Cutting; and Chapter 13, Catherine Lavelle for the subsection on the paediatric liaison CAMHS team.

All specific references to the Scottish administrative and legal systems were contributed by Dr Michael van Beinum.

Contributors

Tricia Brennan, MBChB, DCH, FRCP, FRCPCH, FCEM, is Consultant Paediatrician and Named Doctor for Child Protection for the Sheffield Children's NHS Foundation Trust, and Designated Doctor for Child Protection for Sheffield.

Josie Brown, MBChB, DRCOG, MRCPsych, is Consultant Child and Adolescent Psychiatrist, Southampton General Hospital.

Helen Bruce, FRCPsych, is Consultant Child and Adolescent Psychiatrist, East London NHS Foundation Trust, and Honorary Senior Clinical Lecturer, Barts and the London School of Medicine and Dentistry.

Lois Colling, BSc, MRCPsych, Islington Primary Care Trust, London.

Paul Gill, MBBS, MRCPsych, is Consultant in Liaison Psychiatry, Sheffield Health and Social Care NHSFT, The Longley Centre, Sheffield.

Diana Hulbert, BSc, MBBS, FRCS (Glas.), FCEM, is Emergency Medicine Consultant, Department of Emergency Medicine, Southampton University Hospitals NHS Trust

Tony Kaplan, MBChB, FRCPsych, Cert. Adv. Family Therapy (Sheldon Fellow), Dip. Clin. Hypnosis (UCL), is Consultant Child and Adolescent Psychiatrist at the New Beginning Young People's Crisis Recovery Unit, North London, part of the Barnet, Enfield and Haringey Mental Health Trust.

Ian Maconochie, FRCPCH, FCEM, FRCPI, PhD, is Consultant Paediatrician in the Paediatric Emergency Department, Imperial Academic Health Sciences Centre, London.

Begum Maitra, MBBS, DPM, MRCPsych, MD (Psychiatry), is Consultant Child and Adolescent Psychiatrist, and Jungian Analyst in the East London NHS Foundation Trust (City and Hackney).

Mary Mitchell, MA, BM, MRCPsych, is Consultant Child and Adolescent Psychiatrist, Leigh House Hospital, Winchester, part of the Hampshire Partnership NHS Trust.

Annie Souter, CQSW Social Work, Dip. Social Work, Dip. Family Support and Child Protection, is Team Manager, Children's Social Care, Islington Children's Services, Whittington Hospital, London.

Eric Taylor, MA, MB, FRCP, FMedSci, is Emeritus Professor, Institute of Psychiatry, King's College London.

Avril Washington, MBBS, MRCP, FRCPCH, is Consultant Paediatrician, Homerton University Hospital Foundation Trust.

Abbreviations

ADHD	attention-deficit hyperactivity disorder
CAMHS	child and adolescent mental health services
CBT	cognitive–behavioural therapy
CRB	Criminal Records Bureau
GCS	Glasgow Coma Scale
GP	general practitioner
NHS	National Health Service
NICE	National Institute for Health and Clinical Excellence
NSF	National Service Framework
PMETB	Postgraduate Medical Education and Training Board
PTSD	post-traumatic stress disorder
SIGN	Scottish Intercollegiate Guidelines Network
SSRI	selective serotonin reuptake inhibitor

Tables, boxes and figures

Figures

CHAPTER 1

Introduction

Tony Kaplan

At some point, one in five children and adolescents in the UK will suffer distress or disorganisation of their behaviour sufficient to be considered 'disordered' (Office for National Statistics, 2005). Much of this 'disorder' will be dealt with informally and resolve or persist at a low level, accumulating over time to present at a later stage. Some children and adolescents will be dealt with by various professionals in various capacities – teachers, school nurses, general practitioners (GPs), social workers – and never come to the attention of 'specialists'. Some will be helped by child and adolescent mental health services (CAMHS), without ever needing hospital services. However, some children and adolescents will present at an emergency department in a crisis, they and their families and carers fraught with anguish, expecting the professionals they encounter to have the answers to make things better. Yet what they often encounter is a service stretched to capacity, staff trying to get the job done within a strictly limited time frame, with limited experience of and training in child and adolescent mental health problems and a lack of clarity over what can be done and how to get it done.

This book may contribute to improving and expanding the understanding, knowledge and skills of all practitioners in or called into the emergency department to deal with a child or adolescent with a mental health crisis, and so help them provide a better service to these young people and their families, and afford these young patients and their families a better and more useful experience at a time of crisis.

How big is the problem?

Five per cent of adults attending the emergency department present with significant mental health problems. There are no comparable figures for children and adolescents in the UK, but in the USA studies show a similar proportion of children and adolescents (1 in 20) presenting to emergency departments with mental health-related problems (Thomas, 2003). They point to an increasing use of the emergency department for the emergency assessment of psycho-emotional and behaviour-related problems – between 1995 and 1999, while general paediatric attendance increased by 2%, child and adolescent mental health referrals increased by 60%. Thomas (2003) suggests that the increases are attributed to the greater knowledge of mental health problems in children and adolescents, and hence a greater demand for services, and to the increase in self-harm among teenagers.

The start of a solution

In 2003, the Child and Adolescent Faculty of the Royal College of Psychiatrists set up a working group of interested child psychiatrists, who worked with representatives from the Royal College of Paediatrics and Child Health, the British Association of Emergency Medicine (later the College of Emergency Medicine) and the Royal College of Psychiatrists' Faculty of Liaison Psychiatry, to produce a document examining these problems and possible solutions (Appendix I).

Arising from the deliberations of the working group, there was a request from all parties for a handbook on child and adolescent mental health, adapted for use in the emergency department to act as a user-friendly brief reference book, a practical practice guide and a training resource.

Who is this book for?

This book is written accordingly for anyone who deals with children, adolescents and their families who present in the emergency department with a mental health-related problem or set of problems. It is for first-line practitioners, for their seniors who will consult with them, for their teachers and trainers who will help them develop their skills and knowledge, and for the heads of departments, managers and commissioners required to work together to provide effective and efficient services to meet the needs of this underprovided for group of patients.

What is this book for?

For front-line practitioners we set out what you are expected to know and be able to do (your knowledge base and necessary skills), according to your role and the limits of your responsibility. We set that in a plexus of professional colleagues, disciplines, departments, services and agencies, each with their own competencies, responsibilities and limitations. This will help you 'know the territory', so that when you don't know what to do next, you will know who can advise you and, when your responsibility is exceeded, who to refer on to and how to do that most efficiently and expeditiously. We provide a basic framework of knowledge and practice guidance, which should help you feel and be competent up to the threshold of your responsibility.

For teachers and trainers we provide sufficient information for the training of doctors and other first-line practitioners in the emergency department who will have to deal with young patients with mental health problems, and their families. We leave you to judge the level of competence you wish your trainee to acquire, and to select from this resource accordingly.

For senior professionals and managers we have included a section on the organisation and planning of services, and for commissioners a subsection to help to identify components of services that need to be in place to meet the needs of these children and adolescents, and to determine quality standards for these services.

Why do children and adolescents with mental health-related problems go to the emergency department?

Children and adolescents present to the emergency department when their actions, their behaviour or the way they appear to be suffering becomes intolerable to the people who feel responsible for caring for them. The situation becomes intolerable when it is too upsetting, too frightening or too confusing to be coped with by the physical and emotional resources of the young person and their family and/or other support systems.

The problems that bring children and adolescents to the emergency department may have arisen suddenly and surprisingly (an acute problem), or may be the culmination of a gradual accretion of (chronic) dysfunction with a final precipitant, or the (acute-on-chronic) recurrence of known problems.

What types of problems are there?

Children and adolescents may present with the following.

- Self-harm (this is by far the most common problem presenting to CAMHS).
- Acute psychiatric disorder, which cannot be coped with by carer and cannot be managed by normal out-patient services, including:
  - depression (e.g. because of suicidality, self-neglect, agitation or starvation);
  - psychosis (e.g. because of overwhelmingly high arousal, fear, distress, aggression or unpredictability, or because of bizarre, socially embarrassing or risk-taking behaviour);
  - anxiety syndromes (e.g. because of panic symptoms, insomnia, exhausting demands for reassurance and emotional support, or overwhelming, intrusive mental symptoms (as part of obsessive–compulsive disorder or post-traumatic stress disorder (PTSD));
  - hypomania (e.g. with disinhibition, over-activity).

- Acute exacerbations of behavioural symptoms associated with chronic developmental disorder:
  - autism-spectrum disorders (e.g. insomnia, aggression/frustration reactions);
  - attention-deficit hyperactivity (hyperkinetic) disorders (risk or injuries related to dangerous impulsivity, overwhelming over-activity related to social/environmental context).
- Eating disorders (especially because of medical complications, e.g. fainting, weakness, coldness).
- Delirium, confusional and toxic states.
- Complications of drug/substance/alcohol misuse or withdrawal, including unconsciousness, psychosis, anxiety, behavioural dyscontrol.
- Side-effects of psychotropic medications.
- Medically unexplained symptoms (psychosomatic/conversion symptoms).
- Signs or reports of abuse, including factitious disorders by proxy and/ or neglect.
- Children may also present when their parent is the referred or identified patient, for example a parent presenting with a serious mental illness or where the parent is the victim of domestic violence.
- Behaviour problems, especially violence – when there is no other obvious place for the carers to get help from, or because there is a previous involvement with the hospital (e.g. previous referrals or admissions to paediatrics) and/or a CAMHS history.

What do we know about presenting problems?

In a paper by Behar & Shrier (1995), the most common diagnosis at presentation in an US sample was adjustment disorder (40%), followed by disruptive behaviour disorder (21%), psychotic disorder (12%) and mood disorder (8%). In what is the only UK study of CAMHS presentations to the emergency department, Healy et al (2002) surveyed 107 consecutive emergency attenders at their inner-city emergency service (which included the emergency department of a London teaching hospital). Self-harm was the main presenting problem in a third of the sample. Most of these cases were young girls. After specialist assessment (and brief intervention), most were not admitted for further treatment but were seen for urgent follow-up (75% within 2 weeks) in out-patients, where possible by the same assessing CAMHS professional who had carried out the emergency assessment. Of the attenders who did not self-harm, the most common problem was psychosis, including hypomania (a third of this group), followed by adjustment and other anxiety-related disorders, and problems related to intellectual difficulties. Also seen were problems related to conduct, drug and alcohol misuse, and depression (without self-harm). In this latter group, 5 out of

32 attenders had no psychiatric problems as such. Two-thirds presented out of hours, but no differences from those attending during normal working hours were discerned. Almost two-thirds of all cases had had some previous involvement with CAMHS (48%) and/or Social Services. Healy *et al* (2002) advocate the development of a systematic clinical screening tool for emergency department clinicians to include known psychosocial risk factors (e.g. domestic violence and parental mental illness, the two most common risk factors in their sample), a 'treatment model' (Allen, 1996) for assessment and intervention, and the availability of urgent follow-up, where possible by the same professional involved in the assessment and initial intervention (Greenfield *et al*, 1995) and which is part of an integrated multi-agency approach. A review of the literature on self-harm in young people suggested that over 90% of young people presenting with self-harm at emergency departments fulfilled criteria for a mental health disorder with significant impairment (Skegg, 2005).

How do young people get to the emergency department?

Self-referral (older adolescents only)

When an adolescent presents to the emergency department without their parent(s), other than working out what the problem is and doing something to resolve it, practitioners will also need to know: whether the person is 'competent' ('has capacity') to give or withhold consent for treatment or admission; the limits of confidentiality; how to explore the adolescent's care and support system, and how to exploit this – who to contact or with whom to put them in contact to get help.

Non-professional referrers/escorts

These include parents (most commonly) as well as non-parental carers (e.g. other relatives, foster parents) and friends (in the case of older adolescents).

In dealing with this group of non-professional referrers, the practitioner will also need to understand the nature and limits of parental responsibility (who has it and who doesn't) as this applies to consent and confidentiality, the patterns of care-giving behaviour in those close to the patient, and how to enlist their support in dealing with the child or adolescent.

Professional referrers

- GPs/primary care practitioners
- Paramedics/ambulance crews
- Community CAMHS
- Community paediatric and child health services
- Social Services – area team/duty team, residential/fostering

- Schools and colleges (including school nurses)
- Police

Professional referrers will refer in to the emergency department when their assessment of risk suggests that the young patient needs to be contained safely (i.e. they are explicitly or implicitly requesting admission to a hospital bed) or they need a second opinion or expert view urgently on some aspect of medical management.

This book will help practitioners also understand the nature and presentations of mental health problems in children and adolescents, sufficient to make a risk assessment and risk management plan (which may or may not include hospitalisation), a preliminary crisis intervention and/or to refer on to or consult more expert professionals more effectively where necessary.

How are services currently organised?

There is a great diversity in the delivery of CAMHS emergency services in the UK. Emergency departments are one of a range of provisions that address the needs of children, adolescents and families with acute bio-psychosocial problems. Some areas will have specialised paediatric emergency departments. Some will have primary care out-of-hours assessment centres. Others will have specialised mental health emergency and assessment centres, catering almost exclusively for adults, although some may see young people over the age of 16. There has been a growth in crisis intervention outreach/home-visiting services in line with the National Institute for Health and Clinical Excellence (NICE) guidelines on early intervention. Some areas will have drop-in crisis services, largely provided by voluntary sector organisations.

The provision of specialist services within the emergency department is also variable. A recent review of children's hospital services by the Healthcare Commission for England found that 28% of services were performing poorly with regard to emergency provision (Healthcare Commission, 2006). This diversity and inequity, and the discrepancy between national policy documents, such as the National Service Framework (NSF) (Department of Health, 2004) which applies to England only and the differences in the statutory framework across countries in the UK, makes it impossible to have a set of prescriptions that will apply to all services. Ultimately, local provision is at best a compromise between good practice and the pragmatics of current budgets (often starting from a very low resource base) and the service development trajectory.

The Thomas Coram Research Unit carried out a scoping study of the different ways in which CAMHS commissioners and providers in England are providing emergency support to children and young people at times of mental health crisis (Storey & Stratham, 2007). Although many services can meet the NSF'S requirement for a specialist CAMHS assessment within the next working day, most cannot provide a CAMHS assessment and 'disposal' within the 4 h waiting target for emergency department users. Unless the hospital has its own CAMHS liaison team (not a common provision and then only during working hours almost exclusively), urgent assessment within this time frame is usually provided by paediatric doctors or liaison nurses for under-16-year-olds, and by psychiatry trainees for 16- and 17-year-olds, in some cases aided by crisis teams or in some centres during working hours by adult mental health liaison teams. In some better resourced centres (mainly in relation to teaching hospitals), a CAMHS specialist registrar is available for urgent assessments out of hours, but more commonly there is no CAMHS specialist available for emergency assessments, or the CAMHS specialist registrar provides a secondary assessment after referral from one of the above-mentioned doctors or services.

The Joint Colleges' Working Group on CAMHS in the emergency department are conducting a survey of all emergency departments in the UK to establish the level of CAMHS provision and training in these departments.

Assessing children and adolescents: what's different?

The biggest differences in considering the needs of children and adolescents with mental health, emotional and behavioural difficulties presenting to the emergency department compared with adults are the statutory and social care responsibilities that surround them. Thus, it is vital that practitioners have an understanding of:

- the nature of parental responsibility;
- the child protection framework;
- issues of competency to give consent to or to withhold treatment;
- the rights to confidentiality, consideration and understanding of the family and social support environment into which the young person may be discharged;
- the child's development (the younger the child, the more likely they are to be influenced by changes in family relationships and atmosphere).

Furthermore, assessors will need to bear in mind that the behavioural and emotional state of children and adolescents is influenced to a greater extent by their family (and social) relationships than is the case with adults. A corollary of this is that children's emotional and behavioural problems may exceed the parents' capacity to cope as a consequence of impairments in the adults' functioning, rather than by an escalation in the child's behaviour. These things often go together, interacting in a mutually reinforcing circular causality (e.g. Gutterman *et al*, 1993; Pumariega & Winters, 2003). Thus, the relationship with the parent(s)/carer(s) and their coping style, capacity and resources also need to be included in the assessment of the child.

There is a particular responsibility on those assessing children and adolescents in the emergency department. Thomas (2003) points out that

7

'psychiatric emergency services are brief windows of time in which the child or adolescent and the family are coming (often) for the first time, ready to receive help and engage in change'. The young people or families who present to the emergency department may well not present to services in more routine and ordinary ways, at least not with the drive to resolution, the enhanced motivation usually inherent in a crisis. The intervention they receive in the emergency department may be a unique opportunity for change to the benefit of the child or adolescent, unavailable (or limited) in other settings. As Thomas puts it, 'while the child's ecological context influences the time, nature and severity of the crisis, the organisation of emergency mental health services in the ecology of a healthcare system may influence the outcome of the crisis'.

There are often different organising assumptions and expectations regarding the assessment of paediatric medical patients and the assessment of children and adolescents with mental health problems. The expectation for most general paediatric patients is that the problem(s) leading to attendance at the emergency department may well be able to be resolved effectively by brief treatment and discharge to out-patient care. Child and adolescent mental health presentations in crisis in the emergency department are often met with minimisation of the problem to justify discharge, or the presumption that separation from their family (by admission to hospital) is the default solution, in the short term at least. To some extent this dichotomy arises because most first-line professional staff who see children, adolescents and their families for mental health crisis in the emergency department are relatively untrained. They are not usually able to include in their assessment an understanding of cognitive and emotional development, family/systemic dynamic influences of the child, and even the significance of certain symptoms in the child. Thus, there is a bias to admit children and adolescents for further assessment by a suitably qualified CAMHS professional within the next working day. The tendency is to assess for admission or discharge, 'screening' patients, with an emphasis on examining for pathognomonic indicators and overt presenting symptoms, so as to inform risk management. It is easier in that context to admit than to discharge. It is probably safe to say that little attention is given to crisis intervention to produce change that would limit risk, de-escalate crisis and enhance support that may produce dramatic and fundamental change in the young person's support structures. (That is not to say that admission to hospital also is wrong or disadvantageous.)

Attitudes to CAMHS in the emergency department: what needs to change?

Perhaps because of the lack of training, historically the American experience has been that 'the atmosphere towards psychiatric patients is often negative and hostile. The problems of the children and family are perceived as self-inflicted, deserved outcomes that are evidence of weak, disorganised families, making poor life choices' (Thomas, 2003). The NICE guidelines on self-harm (National Institute for Health and Clinical Excellence, 2004) suggest that this attitude, at least with regard to self-harm, is prevalent in UK hospitals also. There is little research on how decisions are made in the emergency department regarding young people with mental health problems, how this is influenced by the different levels of tolerance in different parents and assessing professionals, or the application of specific threshold criteria within care pathways, nor much research on the negative effects of hospitalisation for young people. Furthermore, recent research by the Mental Health Foundation (2006) on the views of service provision by young people who had self-harmed indicated that young people themselves found emergency department service provision the least helpful, and much preferred low-key community-based help and support. It is therefore not surprising that a community-based questionnaire survey in England indicated that although around 7% of young people aged 15–16 years had self-harmed in the past year, only 12.6% of these young people had gone to an emergency department to seek further help (Hawton *et al*, 2002).

The way forward

The Academy of Medical Royal Colleges (2008), in collaboration with the Department of Health, has issued guidelines and recommendation for service standards and developments to deal with mental health problems across the lifespan presenting to emergency departments. Essentially, for CAMHS, this recommends that CAMHS liaison teams deal with children and adolescents presenting during normal working hours, and that a rota of CAMHS specialists is available to do emergency assessments (and interventions) after hours. In time, this may become the norm. However, for the foreseeable future the solution in most hospitals will be a pragmatic one, based on historical patterns of service delivery and the competing pressures in the local health economy.

The 'Child in Mind' initiative from the Royal College of Paediatrics and Child Health will, over time, produce paediatric trainees who are more aware of and skilled in CAMHS. However, for most children, adolescents and their families with mental health concerns to be better served, practitioners at the front line in emergency departments need to be better trained, more informed and better prepared to take on the challenges that these problems present. This book is our contribution to this part of the solution.

CHAPTER 2

Contextual factors in assessing children and adolescents

Helen Bruce*

Presentation

Children and adolescents change with age in a way that is much more obvious and pronounced than in later life. Children and adolescents, more so than adults, are embedded in and influenced by their family and social systems. The way in which a child or an adolescent presents to the emergency department will be determined in large measure by their stage of psychosocial development and their resultant social and communication skills, and by their family relationships. If there has been a delay in development or difficulties in social and communication skills acquisition, the presentation will be different from that expected for their chronological age. In a situation of fear, unfamiliarity or pain, a child may regress to an earlier stage of development. It is important that the assessor is familiar with developmental processes and the various discontinuities that can occur within them.

Importance of attachment: understanding care-seeking behaviour

The child's attachment behaviour or style emerges from their earliest relationships with their regular carers, usually the parents, and usually most importantly with their mother (in extended family systems this may be another family member). These attachment relationships shape the child's coping style, more explicitly their care-seeking behaviour, in situations of stress or fear. Coming to hospital in an emergency is just the kind of stress that powerfully elicits in the child a need for comfort and protection, and in the carer, feelings of protectiveness engendered by the child's distress. An awareness of attachment will help the assessor make sense of the child's 'illness behaviour', (and their carer's care-giving style),

---

*With special thanks to Tony Kaplan for his contribution (see p. vii).

help to discern the anxieties that underpin this, and allow more sensitive and effective management.

The parent's/carer's behaviour in relation to the child will usually give an indication of how difficult it will be to engage, manage and comfort the child. In a relationship in which the child is securely attached, the child's distress is contained by a response in the carer which is measured (but not necessarily unemotional), empathic, attentive, comforting and protective. Insecure attachments may be apparent in the behaviour of the carer in various ways, and can be categorised into three types. In the first type, the carer is excessively fraught, panicky, angry and/or guilt inducing (in the case of the so-called 'emotionally preoccupied' type). In the second type (the so-called 'avoidant/dismissive' type), the parent/carer is excessively cool and dismissive of the child's distress, minimising their suffering and providing false reassurance. The carer may be judged to be uncaring (unfairly) or insensitive and rigid in their thinking. In the 'unresolved'/'disorganised' type, the parent/carer is chaotic, volatile, vindictive (frightening) and/ or frozen (frightened). This latter type has the greatest correlation with severe mental health problems in the child. The parent may be traumatised, abused or bereaved and in need of help and support to become able to provide adequate parenting, and the child may need protection from their parent's emotionally provocative or abusive behaviour.

Correspondingly, the secure child will more easily be engaged and soothed by healthcare professionals. The insecure anxious, 'ambivalent' child is clingy, untrusting, deeply distressed or even hostile. They will not want to be separated from their carer for assessment or intervention, and will exhibit strong and persistent distress in the face of separation or a feared intervention. However, the presence of the carer may make them more distressed in the face of their own fear of the unknown. This will require patient and sensitive handling to ensure the best outcome on balance. The insecure 'avoidant' child might appear on the surface to be excessively brave, self-reliant and compliant, but they may become aggressive and fiercely oppositional when their usual coping style is overwhelmed, and will have difficulty asking for help, fearing rebuff or humiliation. The insecure 'disorganised' child will appear to be volatile, frozen and/or excessively controlling of others in the face of stress. This pattern is sometimes indicative of child abuse. The motivational conflict inherent in these children and adolescents often leads to contradictory help-seeking behaviour, which is frustrating and confusing to care staff, who may then find themselves unusually filled by reactive feelings of rejection and hostility to the patient.

It is fair to say everyone prefers certainty and agency (the sense of controlling one's environment). A health crisis in a child is frightening and destabilising for most parents. Parents will want information, to be part of all decision-making, and to have their protective relationship with their child recognised and respected. All parents and children, but especially insecurely attached children, adolescents and their reciprocally insecure parents, will have difficulty dealing with uncertainty, and may need repeated explanation (in language they can understand), reassurance and encouragement to feel in control of aspects of the process of intervention that are within their intellectual ability and over which they can safely exercise agency, if only in part. This will help to engage their collaboration, and reduce resistance and opposition.

Importance of the family and other social systems

An exploration and understanding of the child's or adolescent's family and social system will facilitate the identification of the triggering, exacerbating and maintaining factors for the presentation of serious emotional and behavioural problems. The precipitant may, for example, be a crisis in the family, a problem at school (e.g. bullying), a problem in the adolescent's peer group or in a close relationship (e.g. boyfriend/girlfriend), or a combination of these. For example, an adolescent girl self-harmed when the rejection and bullying from her peer group escalated at a time when her mother, who was her usual confidante, became depressed and emotionally unavailable through bereavement, and her favourite teacher went on maternity leave.

The family is, of course, the most important and influential social group for the child up to adolescence, and although thereafter the influence of family relationships has to be balanced against the importance to the adolescent of their peer relationships, it is nevertheless for many still salient. Any rejection, whether explicitly verbalised (e.g. 'I hate you', 'I wish you'd never been born', 'I'm going to have you put in care', 'Go and live with your father then') or inadvertent (e.g. a parent becoming preoccupied by illness, bereavement, divorce or separation, depression, substance misuse, work or other stresses to the exclusion of the child) will be taken to heart by the child, no matter how old they are. This is likely to lead to the child feeling hurt, fearful, sometimes angry, and often sad. Parental illness, disharmony or violence may preoccupy the child, and should form part of the enquiry about the family atmosphere in which the child lives. The child's illness behaviour may be a tactic to bring the parents together or to distract the parent(s) from their own worries or depression. Separations (e.g. during divorce, the estranged parent having reduced contact) or losses (e.g. bereavement of an important family member) will affect the child's sense of security and well-being. Sibling relationships are sometimes implicated in the genesis of the problem, whether through sibling rivalry (of the older towards the younger sibling who is more favoured or protected, or who is catching up quickly mentally or physically; or from the younger to the older sibling who may set standards that seem impossible to attain), overt bullying or abuse, disputes about role (e.g. the oldest boy assuming authority over his older sister as 'the man of the family' after the father leaves) or anticipated displacement after the birth of a new brother or sister. The possibility of child abuse or neglect should always be considered, as these can present covertly in just about every form of emotional and behavioural problem. Of course the family nexus can provide love, warmth, continuity, familiarity and reassurance, and an overwhelming resource for recovery, and this should not be underestimated, and indeed where possible this should be exploited in the child's interest.

Children take social reference from their parents – if, for example, a parent has had a traumatic experience of hospital admission and is accordingly highly anxious during the child's hospital admission, the child will be more anxious than they would otherwise have been. A parent who does not want a young child to divulge family 'secrets' does not have to verbalise this to silence the child. Although families should always be dealt with respectfully, and their wish to comfort and protect their child acknowledged, their presence during all of the assessment of the child may be counterproductive, and their cooperation should be sought, in the interests of the child, to wait separately for a time so the child can be seen on their own. Of course, many parents or other family members are calm and attentive, and their presence can comfort and reassure the child and make the assessment and any interventions much easier. Adolescents should be offered the choice of whether to be seen with or without parents.

During adolescence, young people gradually (or sometimes suddenly and problematically) develop confidence in their capacity to manage on their own without parental guidance. The degree of individuation and autonomy will depend on cognitive maturation, temperament, family dynamic factors, and social and cultural norms and challenges. Adolescents may prefer to confide in friends to sustain their sense of independence, and thus friendships may be very important and more strongly bonded than adults may assume. Disruption of these relationships may have what seems to be a disproportionate effect on the young person's emotional well-being, confidence and sense of self-worth. An acute health or mental health problem and presentation to the emergency department may severely challenge the adolescent's emerging sense of autonomy, and elicit dependency feelings in relation to their parents which may feel shaming. This aspect of an adolescent's relationship with their parents in the emergency department needs careful, sensitive and respectful handling.

Diversity

The family's class, culture, ethnicity and religion need to be considered (see Chapter 9). Beliefs about illness, and especially mental illness, vary across cultures. Illness behaviour may be different, for example the much higher rates of somatisation in situations of emotional stress in some cultures. Beliefs about spirit possession may be a way of describing psychosis in some groups. The stigma of mental illness varies across cultures. Abusive treatment of the child is never acceptable whatever the cultural or religious beliefs, although where certain practices are common and condoned, the child might feel less abused. The assessor should never assume that strange practices are 'normal' for the culture, just because the family are not from the dominant culture. Children of refugee families present other challenges, and the prevalence of post-traumatic reaction is high in both children and parents. They are often unfamiliar with healthcare services and expectations of healthcare professionals. The use of interpreters is essential for children and their families where English is not their first language. Children should not be expected to interpret for their parents. A non-related interpreter should be used when it is important to discuss matters that are confidential to the child or adolescent. This is especially the case where abuse is suspected.

Developmental considerations

Language and comprehension

Self-evidently, the younger the child, the more restricted their vocabulary, less sophisticated their grasp of syntax and more limited their capacity to hold on to and remember bits of information, even when they understand these separately. It is sometimes difficult for professionals untrained in dealing with and unseasoned in the practice of talking to young children, to find the right words or terms to question or to explain something to a young child. Parents or others who know the child well will have a better understanding of the child's language level and be able to couch things in a way the child can understand. They can act as 'interpreters' where necessary. However, where possible, the practitioner should talk directly to the child – this will convey interest and care, and be more reassuring to the child than a practitioner who does not seem equipped or motivated to talk to a child in 'child-friendly' way. When uncertain, the practitioner should err on the side of simplification, using simple words and uncomplicated, short sentences, without an unnecessarily infantilising tone, which may be humiliating or disconcerting to a more competent child.

Competence

The issue of competence to give or withhold consent should always form part of the assessment at every contact with healthcare staff. Competence (or capacity) is a judgement made by clinical assessment and in relation to the specific decision to be made. Consent, capacity and the legal framework for children and adolescents is fully discussed in Chapter 7.

It should also be remembered that consent is essential before information is sought from or disclosed to a third party.

Developmental psychopathology

Children under 5 years

It is relatively uncommon for children under 5 years to present to the emergency department with emotional or behavioural problems. In this age group, children may present with regulatory problems (e.g. sleeping and feeding problems), or when the parent has become exhausted because the child won't stop crying or having extreme tantrums. In these cases, the circumstances and distress of the parents must be carefully considered; underlying exacerbating factors may exist in the family or with the parents' own mental health or ability to cope.

A crisis presentation in a very young child will often have its basis in a family or parental crisis. Children may present as a direct result of parental illness, for example in a case of post-partum depression, where there are risks for the development of insecure attachment and dysregulation of the infant. Assessment should give importance to the needs of the family and parents and what stresses they are facing, the social situation of the family and what support is available to them, both informally and from professionals.

Children in this age group may present with psychological aspects of medical disorders or with psychological aspects of specific sensory impairments. An example of this would be sleep disorders associated with gastric reflux or painful juvenile arthritis. A chronic medical condition may result in repeated episodes of hospitalisation disrupting the formation and development of secure attachment relationships.

Children under 5 can also present in the emergency department with behavioural problems due to underlying autism or attention-deficit hyperactivity disorder (ADHD), although this is more commonly recognisable in the 5- to 11-year age group, as described below, and for this to be the presenting problem as an emergency implies that there are background factors that have made the parents less able to cope, as above.

Importantly, children in this age group may also be seen when there is suspicion of, or actual, abuse. The most common presentation to the emergency department of children under 5 who will require a psychosocial intervention is a 'non-accidental' injury.

Children 5–11 years

In this middle childhood group there will be a decline in presentation of the regulatory disorders, but an increasing presentation of challenging behaviours associated with underlying neurodevelopmental disorders. The most common presentations include behaviour disorders, adjustment disorders, psychosomatic problems and difficulties secondary to a medical illness. In this group, as has been described above, for the family to present to the emergency department in crisis, an incident will usually have provoked a crisis in an already overstretched family network and the parents having reached the end of their ability to cope with the child's difficulties.

Parents may bring children who have ADHD or who are on the autism spectrum to the emergency department because of their apparently uncontrollable challenging behaviours. An incident, for example being excluded from school following an aggressive assault on another child, may well underlie the presentation at that particular time and care needs to be taken to elicit such incidents in history taking.

Acute stress or a very stressful life event in a child in this age group may result in a short-lived stress reaction, an adjustment disorder or PTSD, and the child may be presented in crisis to the emergency department, with distressing fears, disordered sleep with persistent nightmares or night terrors, or psychosomatic symptoms.

Less commonly, there may be presentations with severe anxiety, obsessive–compulsive disorders, affective disorders and self-harm. These groups of conditions become more common as the child grows into adolescence, and in this last age group are more likely to present to community services rather than to the emergency department.

Adolescents 12–18 years

Adolescents differ from the younger age groups in that they are less dependent on their parents and family and have more autonomy. Challenging behaviours are more difficult to contain in adolescents because of their increasing size and strength compared with younger children. They also have more access to and are more likely to engage in risk-taking behaviours. Adolescents may well present to the emergency department with peers rather than with family members. It is particularly common for adolescent girls to present with a female friend rather than a parent.

In the adolescent age group, the whole range of 'adult-type' mental health problems may present, but sometimes have different antecedents and be expressed slightly differently according to the psychosocial developmental stage and life-cycle changes and challenges, compared with presentations seen in adult populations.

The most common presentation is self-harm. The assessment of self-harm in adolescence resembles that of an adult mental health assessment for self-harm, but the influences of family, school and peer group are an important part of the assessment. In this age-group especially, self-harm has to be seen in its developmental context. It is often an attempted resolution of a motivational conflict around continuing dependence and the wish for greater independence – the adolescent is ashamed to feel reliant on sources of emotional support they feel they should have outgrown, or the person giving emotional support has become more distant and inaccessible, or overtly rejecting. Self-harm becomes the adolescent's way of showing anger towards the person to whom they feel emotionally dependent, without driving them away, eliciting both guilt (the carer is made to feel attacked as neglectful), protectiveness and heightened attachment.

An adolescent may present with the first episode of an acute psychotic episode. The adult forms of the common psychoses may become evident in adolescence, although often in the early episodes the symptoms are less clear and delusions less systematised. Cannabis use is a common concomitant, but it is not always clear whether this is a coincidental finding (cannabis smoking is common among teenagers), a precipitant or a causative agent. Often in this age group, because of lifestyle or subcultural congruence, warning signs may have been ignored and the first presentation to mental health services is via the emergency department. This may be the case for other mental health crises such as severe mood disorders. In severe mental illness presentations, the mental state examination will resemble that done in adult mental health services.

Increasingly in this age group, intoxication with drugs or alcohol may also present acutely to the emergency department.

Anorexia nervosa becomes more common in adolescence, and attendance in the emergency department may result from medical complications of the young person's eating disorder.

Adolescents may present with issues of underlying abuse – sexual, emotional or physical. Emergency department staff need to be alert to this possibility, as abuse issues can present in a multitude of different ways, most importantly including self-harm and psychosomatic problems. Indeed, self-harm is the most common initial presentation of sexual abuse in this age group.

Because of the increased risk to others and because the child is now bigger and stronger, violence as part of a conduct disorder, with or without ADHD or the autism-spectrum disorder, may lead to an adolescent being brought to the emergency department.

Special consideration needs to be given to adolescents who have reached the transition phase into adult services. At this point there is often a discontinuity of care and service provision, and this can lead to a crisis presentation for the adolescent, who has been left temporarily without the professional support they had previously depended on.

Assessment of children and adolescents

Seeing the patient with and/or without the parent(s)

The assessing healthcare professional will need to decide whether to interview the child or adolescent together with their carers or on their own. A sequential combination is usually recommended, although it is not always clear whether to start with the young person alone or with the parent present. For younger children, it is more usual to start with the parent present; indeed, usually this will only be possible with the parent/caregiver present. If abuse is suspected, it is vital that the child is seen separately, although if the child can be admitted to a paediatric ward this can be delayed and left to a more experienced and senior colleague once the child is settled (child protection procedures must be initiated nevertheless). Adolescents may well prefer to be interviewed alone and may insist on this. It may still be important to see them together with their carers, both to observe the quality of their relationship and to enhance communication (a deficit in which may have contributed to the adolescent's vulnerability). It is always important whatever the age or developmental stage to talk to the young person and include them as much as possible in the assessment process.

Collateral history

It is essential to take a collateral history from the carers/parents, as well as from any professionals who have been involved in the patient's care.

Legal responsibility

It is important to establish who has parental responsibility for the child. Married parents of the child both have parental responsibility unless this has been removed from them legally (e.g. in adoption proceedings). If the parents are unmarried (and the father is not named on the birth certificate), the father only has parental responsibility if this has been formally and legally granted – it is not assumed. If the child is in public care, the Local Authority (via Social Services) shares parental responsibility with the parent(s) if the child is on a full or interim care order, but the Local Authority has no parental responsibility if the child is merely 'accommodated' under Section 20 of the Children Act 1989. No other carer has parental responsibility even if the child lives with them (e.g. foster parents, residential social workers, other relatives), unless they have a residence order made out to them (see Chapter 7).

Child protection register

A system should be in place to alert staff if children and adolescents presenting to the emergency department are recorded on what used to be the local child protection register (now the 'list of children') who are the subject of a child protection plan. The list should be present in or at least accessible to the emergency department and gives an indication of any current child abuse and neglect concerns. Under new guidance, the children listed are those who are still considered to be at risk of significant harm, and not those who were harmed previously but later, when circumstances changed, considered to be safe. However, the register lists only children registered in the local borough, so this safeguard only applies where the hospital is in the same borough in which the concerns have been recorded. Absence from the register does not mean the child has never been abused.

CHAPTER 3

Emergency assessment and crisis intervention

Tony Kaplan

The nature of crisis

Crisis is an opportunity for rapid, meaningful and positive change, where change has not been possible before. Because the stakes are heightened, individuals are more amenable to change or compromise than usual, and the unfamiliar circumstances allow 'thinking outside the box', the co-creation or acceptance of new solutions for people who may be set in their ways with rigid or restricted coping preferences. Some of the people who present in crisis to the emergency department will not seek help from conventional sources or not seek help in conventional ways (because of their social inhibition, isolation, shame or fear, or because their belief systems, derived from cultural heritage or family myth or experience disallow this). Some will have limited access to healthcare. Presentation to the emergency department may be a rare opportunity to engage them and thereby to make a significant difference to the life of the child or adolescent (and their family).

Crisis intervention

Crisis intervention starts knowingly or unknowingly from the moment of first contact, and occurs cumulatively as the patient and family move through the different disciplines and teams they are required to encounter on their way to a resolution.

The purpose of crisis intervention in the emergency department is:

- to effect recovery and thus discharge;
- to produce sufficient amelioration to allow discharge;
- to provide containment of anxiety or behavioural problems to enable further more specialist assessment to occur;
- to negotiate admission.

Unless overridden by protocols in your department, the outcome will depend on the inherent resources of the young person and their support system, the power of the intervention (or set of interventions) relative to the stresses, and the resultant appraisal of outcome (the risk assessment). Ideally, the 'disposal' (admission, discharge or referral on) should occur after the initial intervention, not after the initial assessment only.

What is assessment for?

Assessment informs and contributes to:

- the initial intervention (to see what can change);
- an accurate risk assessment, taking into account the outcome of the initial intervention(s);
- the formulation of a robust risk management plan;
- the care and treatment plans (or the referral on).

To make an assessment with all these in mind, it is important that the presenting problem is well understood in terms of its nature, its genesis, its determinants and mediators, and its function(s).

What type and standard of assessment you will be expected to make will depend on the organisation of your department, protocols in place, the resources at your disposal, and the availability of more specialists to refer on to. The curricula of training for paediatric and child health doctors, emergency medicine doctors and psychiatrists all require the acquisition of the skills and knowledge to make a mental health assessment of a child or adolescent. In some hospitals, referral on to the 'experts' in the required field happens quickly and efficiently. However, because some hospitals are less well resourced, a less 'expert' doctor or another member of the clinical team will be required to make the assessment in some cases. With the contraction of paediatric beds as a consequence of the growth and development of ambulatory child health services, and the change in the law that hitherto has restricted the young person's right to refuse admission and treatment, it is likely the practice of automatically admitting young people with mental health problems to paediatric beds for further specialist assessment the next day will be challenged more often. This will then require more rigorous assessment in the emergency department and the ability of the assessing team(s) to provide crisis interventions that will reduce risk and morbidity.

Some of what follows in this chapter may seem too specialist, but you may wish to learn the assessment and intervention techniques described out of interest to deepen your understanding of the problems you will encounter, to advance your skills and your job satisfaction (helping people change is very satisfying), or simply because one day there will be no one to refer on to and you will need to know how to assess and intervene competently and safely to avoid the patient's crisis becoming your crisis. Of course, even if there is no one to refer on to in an emergency, in most services there is someone available to offer specialist consultation and advice. The more you know and the more competent you are at intervening, the more useful this consultation will be.

Understanding the presenting problem

How the presenting problem arises

All people, but especially children and adolescents, exist in social support systems. These systems include the family, the extended family, other carers, friends and friendship groups, other significant adults (e.g. teachers or work supervisors), and the established caring professionals and agencies that know the child or adolescent. Up to the presentation to emergency services, it can be presumed that the supportive components of these systems are working well enough together to buffer the child or adolescent against the stresses they are under to allow them to endure their adversity, albeit with a degree of discomfort.

Other than when there are inherent organic factors underlying the mental illness, the young person presents to the emergency department with a mental health problem when:

- they are overwhelmed by a sudden and unexpected extreme stress or loss (a traumatic event);
- they experience a new stress or a sudden increase in an existing stress (a precipitant) which is added to existing accumulated (underlying) stresses, to the extent that the resources of the young person and the support systems are overwhelmed;
- they find the support they have relied on to keep them functioning well enough is reduced – there is a change in the support system which destabilises the balance of the components of the system that are mutually dependent (e.g. the mother becomes ill or depressed, the therapist goes on holiday, there is an unexpected change of social worker, school ends) and there is no (planned) alternative support in place, and what the young person then does to invite compensatory care from someone else in the system or from a new system fails;
- the attempt to restore or re-impose a strategy of coping which no longer 'fits' or to re-organise the system to work better produces more strain (e.g. a child finds that increasing the emotional demands on their mother, something that distracted her from her worries previously, makes her more depressed and withdrawn; inviting the involvement of an estranged father in the hope of supporting the mother provokes rejection by the mother because of perceived disloyalty);
- the child or adolescent feels they cannot ask in a straightforward way for support or comfort from the person they most want this from (because they expect an angry rebuff, humiliation or disinterest, or because they don't wish to add to that person's burden);
- a combination of any of the above.

The result is symptomatic illness and/or illness behaviour, the reflex or instinctive behaviour that accompanies or mimics illness to elicit care necessary to restore health and well-being, and to reset the equilibrium in the system.

Who presents?

Part of the nature of social support systems is that people feel responsible for one another, either because this is expected (a social norm), or because they are duty bound (by contract or under the law) or because they care. Where children and young people are concerned, this is even more the case. Young people may present themselves to the emergency department for help to restore their health or coping sufficiently to try to manage again independently in the community, to seek shelter and comfort when they have none accessible, or to elicit care by proxy (their parents or carers will be alerted to their distress). But more usually, they are brought in to the emergency department by caring others, and usually by people who are, or at least feel, responsible for them. It is when the people with responsibility for the child's or young person's safety and well-being can no longer cope (they feel too much anxiety, distress, anger, fear, confusion) with how the child or young person with mental health problems is behaving (what they are doing or how they are being) that they bring them to someone they think can fix them (at best), or at least make the child or young person bearable to live with and ensure that they are safe while they recover.

Relationship between stress and the presenting problem

Stress interacts with the person's vulnerability (what makes this person less able to cope with this stress – inherent or acquired factors) and their resilience (what makes them more able to cope, be less affected) to produce the (behavioural) outcome – the presenting problem (Fig. 3.1).

Stress

To understand the child's or adolescent's reaction to the stresses they describe and to make predictions about the likely course of their emotional state, it is important to understand the nature of the stress (Box 3.1 and Table 3.1). Stressors may be:

- single, multiple or complex:
    - an example of a single stressor would be a broken leg suffered by a teenager in a road traffic accident;
    - if, in this example, the teenager in question had had another unrelated stress, for example the recent death of a pet, they would have multiple stressors to cope with;

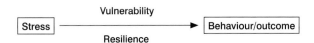

Fig. 3.1 Behavioural outcomes of stress.

Box 3.1 Nature of the stress: practice points

- The first stressor identified is often not the only stressor
- Children and adolescents presenting with mental health problems will usually have multiple or complex stressors
- The effects of the same stressor are different for different children and adolescents
- Stressors need to be examined, not only with regard to the environment the young person comes from, but, importantly, also with regard to the environment they will return to
- Stressors occur in predictable domains in the life of children and adolescents – these should be probed systematically (e.g. 'Do you have any worries about...')

- if the teenager's girlfriend, who usually provided him with emotional support, was seriously injured in the same accident, this would then constitute complex stressors – stressors that interact with one another. In this example, the need for comfort from the girlfriend cannot be met, compounded by concern for the girlfriend's survival, and his blaming himself for her injury with resultant self-punishment, a need to suffer more. The complexity may come from the interaction of the precipitating or immediate stress with an underlying stress, for example, the teenager is struggling with academic work, and worries about the time he will miss from school recovering from his broken limb.
- self-limiting, enduring or intermittent:
  - with self-limiting stressors, once the stress is effected, there is no (predictable) recurrence of that stress – the road traffic accident is a random event; the pet only dies once (of course the effects of the stress on the person may persist, but once it has been coped with, the level of functioning of the young person is stable and an assessment of their functioning then is valid);
  - with enduring stressors, there is no predictable relief from the stress – for example, persistent bullying at school, poverty, overcrowding (if the young person is removed from the stress, their functioning may improve, but predictably if they are to be returned to the stressful environment, their functioning will deteriorate – this has to be factored in as part of the assessment);
  - with intermittent stressors, the recurrence is predictable, but there are times in between that there is relief also – for example, the father who is violent only on weekends when he is drunk.

Vulnerability and resilience

Different people are affected to a different extent by the same stresses. Some will be more affected because their temperament (genetically

Table 3.1 Predictable domains of stress for children and adolescents

Domain	Stressor
Family	Relationships (conflict)
	Health concerns
	Bereavement
	Changes in organisation (separation, divorce, reconstitution)
	Socio-economic (employment, housing, money)
School	Peer relationships (conflict, exclusion, isolation, bullying)
	Relationships with teachers/counsellors/mentors
	Work – exams, course work, specific learning difficulties
Social	Friendships and rivalries
	Romantic relationships
	Sport, activities, interests
	Drugs and alcohol
	Debts
	Gangs

endowed), life experience and deficits in their social support makes them so – this totality is their vulnerability. Some will be less affected, accounted for by their resilience, determined by the same domains.

A stress that is coped with adequately and from which positive lessons are learned is strengthening and contributes to resilience. For example, a boy being chased by a dog jumps over a wall. He learns that: (a) he can run fast; (b) he can think quickly; and (c) being attacked (by a dog) does not lead inevitably to being injured/vanquished. The coping may be partial and the lessons idiosyncratic – for example, a little boy intervenes by shouting to stop his father hitting his mother. The father hits the boy, but leaves the mother. The boy learns that: (a) he can inhibit or overcome his fear and intervene; (b) he can intervene effectively (to stop a catastrophe – his mother being killed); (c) the pain of being hit is not as bad as he thought it would be; and (d) it is compensated for by his mother's pride in him.

A stress that has been overwhelming contributes to vulnerability (to this stress or type of stress) in the future, and this is cumulative – the more the child/adolescent 'fails' (to cope), the more vulnerable they become until they assume they will never succeed ('learned helplessness' – an antecedent of depression). A stress that is not coped with and repeated over time becomes a vulnerability to that stress.

In the emergency department, you will not usually be expected to explore long-term ('distal') vulnerability or resilience, for example, that comes from temperament or early attachment influences, but some will often become apparent, especially in the family domain (Box 3.2).

Box 3.2 Factors contributing to vulnerability and resilience

The most common early/longer-term vulnerability factors to enquire about are:

- the loss of a parent (or significant relative) through death or divorce
- experiencing at an early age parental violence as a witness or victim
- parental mental illness or substance (including of course alcohol) misuse
- any premature sexualised experience
- social dislocation through moving home or country

Recent ('proximal') vulnerability factors that will be important to establish in your assessment include:

- social exclusion or isolation
- academic failure
- chronic victimisation
- chronic physical illness

General protective factors against stress include:

- a reliable relationship with at least one caring adult
- positive, supportive sibling (and peer) relationships
- inherent sources of self-esteem (e.g. sporting prowess)
- higher intelligence and problem-solving ability

Note also

- Asking young people about their strengths and successes will help to counteract demoralisation
- Eliciting their positive coping strategies will help to make them active rather than passive in their style of coping, and this will produce a more favourable outcome in the short term (they will recover more quickly) and in the longer term (they will learn more positive and useful lessons for the future)
- Assessment is, in and of itself, an intervention and produces change

Emergency assessment in practice

Emergency assessment in practice usually goes through a number of steps, including informal, 'process' interventions, the outcome of which informs the next stage (that of risk assessment) and the development of a risk management plan. The non-specific 'process' aspects of assessment (providing emotional containment and managing disorganisation) are the most therapeutic. These are not specific therapeutic skills – these are things professionals dealing with patients in the emergency department do already. How well they do it, of course, varies.

Containment

The first stage is the co-creation of the emotional environment in which the assessment will take place. All individuals learn best in an environment that is calm, warm and stimulating. This is achieved through the interviewer acting as an 'affect modulator' – being calm and patient with over-aroused patients and families, and injecting energy, and even humour, where the patient is withdrawn. Effective therapists transmit a confidence in their ability to be useful (without arrogance or omnipotence – this engenders hope), their warmth, interest and accurate empathy, respect for the patient's uniqueness, and a sense of endeavour and purpose in line with the patient's goals (Box 3.3).

Managing disorganisation

The next stage is the managing of the sense of disorganisation that a crisis invariably evokes. This sense of disorganisation may be internal to the patient – that is, a disorganisation in their thinking and of their usual coping strategies. The disorganisation may be systemic – that is, affecting the way the family and others in the support system work together to offer care and comfort to remedy the problem and to restore equilibrium.

The description below addresses disorganisation at both levels, but will of course depend on whether you are seeing the child/adolescent alone or with their family and carers. Unless there are specific reasons to avoid this (e.g. evident or threatened violence, or a specific request of the patient), there is substantial advantage in seeing the child or adolescent with their parent(s) and/or carer(s), at least at first. (They should also be offered the

---

Box 3.3 Creating a positive environment during assessment

- Be aware of the power of eye contact
- Modulate your voice:
  - to sooth and comfort (but be aware that sounding too sad or sympathetic may make the patient feel worse, at least more passively dependent)
  - to reduce arousal (softer)
  - to increase energy or affective tone (louder)
  - to reassure small children of your benign intentions (raising the pitch of your voice, but not excessively – you should not sound like a chipmunk!)
- Listen actively (restating what has been said, checking what has been said) and open-mindedly (not, at least early on, offering alternative meaning or interpretation, or prematurely offering advice which presumes a 'problem stereotype')
- Offer opportunities for every member of the family to have their say, but not to the exclusion of the patient's point of view: make explicit that you will want to understand each person's point of view, but that understanding the patient's point of view must be your first and overriding concern
- If the atmosphere with family present is too inflammatory, see the patient on their own
- Sit obliquely opposite a paranoid or hostile patient or family member – sitting directly opposite may arouse confrontation

---

opportunity to see a professional on their own if indicated or if they so wish, and this is mandatory if there are child protection concerns.)

Enhancing communication

- Providing a forum for talking and listening
- Providing a fulcrum for conversation – some family members or the patient may find it easier to talk to you and be overheard by the others, than talking directly to one other ('triangulation'), and will allow you, as someone with authority, knowledge and resources, to conduct the conversation – that is, to say who talks when.

Improving coherence

Orderliness

Eliciting information in an organised and systematic way (through the process of formal, semi-structured assessment).

Meaning

Improving the understanding of what is being said by:

- asking for clarification (factual/explicit meaning);
- checking inferences (implicit meaning);
- examining the emotional impact of what is being said;
- exploring the function of what is being said (why is it being said in a particular way/in that tone of voice, for example to be provocative, to elicit sympathy);
- giving factual information (e.g. the meaning of a physical symptom, the options available, the processes involved).

Giving perspective

Of time

Traumatic events and memories are in the past; the future hasn't yet happened – the feared consequence may not happen, plans can change; decisions and actions in the present will influence outcomes in the future.

Of scale

Close to the impact of events, the scale always seems larger – the interviewer may help the patient be realistic about the scale of the misfortune.

Of range

Many people, especially adolescents, in crisis or as an habitual tendency, dichotomise – see things as either/or, good/bad, right/wrong – rather than along a dimension of one thing or another, as a balance of factors. The interviewer can counteract demoralisation or catastrophic expectations by pointing out the spectral variability or asking the patient to scale things numerically on an analogue scale (e.g. how difficult you find that on a scale of 1 to 10).

Establishing the presenting problem

Some generic questions to ask young people towards understanding the presenting problem are listed in Box 3.4. These questions are not appropriate for younger children, but can be adapted with a little imagination, or used to interrogate the presenting problem with the parent(s).

Other problems and stresses

The interviewer should then ask if the young person has other problems or stresses, which might be making life more difficult and making it harder to cope with the first identified (presenting) problem. The sequence of questions in Box 3.4 can be followed for any subsequently identified problems. Stresses that may constitute problems in their own right, or that increase vulnerability, should be probed for systematically through the domains identified earlier.

Establishing background context and influences

Understanding the contexts in which the problems operate and the possible influences of these is important in any comprehensive assessment (Box 3.5).

Principles and purpose of risk assessment

For the assessing professional, the risk evaluation is in effect in two parts: what are the risks in discharging this patient, and what are the risks of admitting this patient? The welfare and safety of the child/adolescent are paramount.

The risks of admission may include:

- disrupting (if only temporarily) the familiar caring environment and support network;
- undermining coping capacity;
- enhancing a passive, dependent coping style;
- exposure (in the case of admission to an in-patient psychiatric setting) to other high-risk children/adolescents and through them learning maladaptive coping behaviour;
- exposure (in in-patient psychiatric settings) to a somewhat unpredictably risky, disturbing and sometimes dangerous environment;
- stigma;
- the risk to other children in the ward.

Risks of discharge may include:

- the condition will get worse if the patient does not have hospital care or if they return to a damaging environment;
- the patient/family are likely to fail to attend for necessary follow-up;
- the patient might be harmed;
- the patient might harm someone else;

Box 3.4 Questions to ask young people about the presenting problem

- What is the problem?
- Who is this a problem for? Is it a problem for you (only) or is it a problem for someone else? In which way?
- Who else is affected by your having the problem?
- Why is this a problem for you? In which way/to what extent is it not 'normal' for you/for anyone your age?
- Have you had this problem before?
- If it has happened more than once, when does it happen (continuous/ongoing, episodic)? How frequently does it happen?
- When doesn't it happen? When doesn't it happen when you're expecting it to happen? *(This alerts the patient to exceptions to the rules about the problem they have constructed for themselves – the exceptions will give information about what the patient is doing inadvertently and probably intuitively to pre-empt the problem, or circumstances that are less provocative and more salubrious, pointing the way to easily accessible solutions.)*
- What makes it worse/more likely to occur?
- What makes it better/less likely to occur?
- How do you know when it's starting? *(This may elucidate triggers, allowing for early intervention in the symptom cycle.)*
- What do you notice when it starts to get better? *(This question puts into the patient's mind the idea of recovery and instils optimism.)*
- What have you tried to do (so far/before/when you last had to deal with something like this) to change things?
- What has helped? (Why not do more of that? Why hasn't that helped this time?)
- What hasn't helped? (Why not – effort, time?)
- Who has tried to help? Who might help? Who has helped before?
- What outcome do you want? What is better/enough?
  - How much does it need to change for you to notice that it is getting better?
  - Is it better to not resolve the problem unless/until you can resolve it completely, or better to resolve the problem a little bit or in stages?
- What would be different in your life if the problem disappeared? What are the advantages of change?
- What would you notice first if you woke up in the morning and the problem had gone away? *(This 'miracle question' often has the effect of lifting the patient's mood and allowing the possibility of a good outcome to enter the patient's imagination.)*
- What might be less good if the problem went away?
  - Who might be worse off?
  - Why might you be better off keeping the problem going for a while? *(E.g. a person with depression may be free from responsibilities and overburdening expectations only while they're 'ill'.)*
- What do you think will help? What can you do differently that will make a positive difference? *(This latter form of question promotes agency and active problem solving.)*
- What help do you want from me/us? *(Again, it's important that this question is framed to invite the young person to actively ask for assistance to achieve their goals, rather than feel decisions are being made for them and solutions imposed on them as if they were passive recipients of care.)*

Box 3.5 Presenting problem: contexts and background

Family
- Composition
    - Parents (get surnames of both)
    - Siblings
    - Extended family – involved?
- Organisation
    - Separation/divorce/reorganisation (i.e. step-parents)
    - Who is living in the home?
- Stresses
    - Relationships
    - Illness
    - Social
- Legal restrictions
    - Court orders
    - Parental responsibility

School/college
- Name
- Type (e.g. mainstream, special needs)
- Contact/informant (e.g. Head of Year? Permission to contact them?)

Other involved agencies
- Social Services
- Child and family mental health services
- Youth offending team

Historical factors and influences
- History of previous illness(es)
- Family history of illness(es)
- Forensic history – involvement with police or courts

Drugs and alcohol use

Early vulnerability and resilience factors
- Developmental history: this is not usually explored in a crisis situation, but early history may emerge from the spontaneous accounts of the young person or family member.

- the patient might seriously harm themselves or even take their own life.

Risk assessment is not static. It changes according to the circumstances that prevail. Thus, the risks at the time of the dangerous act are not necessarily the same at the time of the assessment interview – things may have changed, or been changed, by the process of time or as a consequence of the dangerous act (e.g. the effect on the family's awareness and emotions, which may alter their capacity to provide support).

The risk assessment informs the crisis intervention (at least to set some limit on what outcomes are acceptably safe); but the crisis interventions also inform the risk assessment – the crisis intervention will hopefully reduce (some) risks, or at least give a better sense of how 'stuck' the young person and family are with their difficulties.

Risk factors should be balanced against protective factors (a 'safety assessment').

Risk assessment is cumulative – as the patient passes through the emergency department, each practitioner's risk evaluation informs the risk assessment of the next.

Risk assessment is the business and responsibility of all practitioners in the emergency department, if only to inform risk management to the extent of keeping the patient safe until the next professional in the chain of assessment sees them.

(For a detailed exposition of the risk assessment for suicide, see Chapter 5.)

Crisis intervention

By providing emotional containment and managing disorganisation by the process of assessment hitherto, the practitioner has already provided the initial stages of the crisis intervention. The next stage is goal setting.

Goal setting

Establishing who needs what

This may have been set out and answered partially or in full through the questioning around the presenting problem in relation to the following questions (Box 3.4).

- What do you want in order to cope?
- What has to change for you to feel you can cope?
- What change is good enough (for you to manage for the time being)?
- What do you need to do to get this?
- What do you want/need from others in your support network?
- What do you want from me/our service?

If they have been established already, it is worth reiterating the goals in summary.

Those responsible for the child/adolescent will need to feel that they can cope before they can safely take the child or adolescent home. This can be addressed by reiterating what the responsible adults have said, in relation to the presenting problem, about what they haven't been able to cope with/put up with, and by asking:

- what do you need to see your child doing differently or hear from them that's different enough to feel you could cope with looking after them at home;
- what support (family/friends/other services) will help you to cope?

These questions must be posed and addressed operationally as behaviours that can be observed and verified, especially for this to be effective in addressing anxiety. As an example, if the parent says 'I want my child to be happy', the practitioner may ask 'If your child were happy, what would they be doing that would tell you they were happy, or what would they have stopped doing?'

Negotiations, commitments and working contracts

The young person should then be given the opportunity to negotiate these 'minimum change criteria', and to say whether they think they can meet them (already or in the future), what would help them to meet them, and to establish whether they wish to meet them (if not, why not – the questioning around why having the problem is better than not having it would be fruitful in this case.)

Once these are agreed, summarise and record succinctly, and get or test out the commitment of the 'players' to make these arrangements work and hold. Remind the participants of their motivation to make the necessary changes, i.e. what's in it for them.

Consequences of not achieving the minimum change criteria

One important (agreed) consequence may be admission to hospital (voluntarily or compulsorily if the risks are high enough), or at least an agreement to return to the hospital or attendance at or involvement of other agreed sources of intervention (e.g. Social Services, police).

Risk assessment and management planning

Review risk assessment in light of the crisis intervention outcome(s). Make a risk management care plan and check this is understood and accepted by all. If there is not agreement to proceed safely, then areas of compulsion need delineation – that is, what will have to happen even without the express agreement of all to ensure safety and well-being, and the legal mechanisms that will be employed to ensure this. This, for example, may need addressing in cases requiring child protection interventions, or with young people who are mentally ill or at high risk of suicide who do not comply with the risk management plan, including, if necessary, admission to hospital.

Child and adolescent mental health services follow-up should be offered routinely.

CHAPTER 4

Child and adolescent mental health presentations in the emergency department

Josie Brown*

Depression and self-harm

This is the most common mental health problem or set of problems you will encounter in the emergency department.

Both children and adolescents can become persistently depressed. Common presentations include a (variable) combination of:

- low self-esteem and negative self-image;
- somatic complaints;
- social withdrawal;
- depressed mood;
- marked diminution of or loss of the capacity to enjoy things (anhedonia);
- anxiety (including separation anxiety) and agitation;
- irritability/anger (to self or others)/lowered frustration tolerance;
- loss of appetite (with loss of weight in the more severe form) or increased food intake ('comfort eating');
- sleep problems of various kinds – an anxious child or adolescent with depression may have trouble getting to sleep or be kept awake by depressive ruminations. In the most severe form, the young person wakes early, can't get back to sleep and lies awake with profound feelings of hopelessness; others will want to stay in bed and sleep for long periods;
- suicidal ideation: this is uncommon in pre-pubertal children, but children of this age may express thoughts of, for example, running away or jumping into the middle of the road or out of a window. Suicidal ideation is more common in adolescents with depression, sometimes as a fleeting thought but sometimes as a more formed idea and with clear intention to act on this.

Adolescents with depression may present as an emergency to the emergency department with suicidal thoughts, self-harm, self-mutilation, severe self-neglect, starvation or extreme agitation.

*With special thanks to Lois Colling, Diana Hulbert, Tony Kaplan and Catherine Lavelle for their contributions (see p. vii).

Management

- Remember that marked agitation or withdrawal may indicate someone is significantly depressed.
- Be patient and listen attentively – some children and adolescents with depression will assume that the listener's haste means they are worthless, and will become more withdrawn or defensive and hostile to protect themselves from reflex feelings of rejection. Either of these reactions will make your task more difficult.
- Do not be glib, offer hasty reassurance or minimise the young person's difficulties – this will only make them feel foolish: it will be more effective to acknowledge their distress, recognise that with their depressive cognition life must seem awful and problems difficult to put right, but offer the possibility of alternative viewpoints and solutions, and help them to test these out.
- Take seriously talk of suicide: remember a substantial proportion of people who take their own lives present to medical services shortly beforehand.
- Be aware of covert (undisclosed) self-harm and ask appropriate questions to elicit this information.
- Take corroborative history from a relative or friend if possible.
- If possible, see the young person with their parent(s)/carer(s) for at least part of the interview:
  - to explain or allow the young person to explain their difficulties, the nature of depression, and to help the parent(s)/carer(s) to take this seriously;
  - to help you gauge whether the family home is likely to be a safe and supportive environment to discharge the young person into, or whether the home environment and family relationships may undermine an already precarious adjustment and tip the patient into a suicidal state or aggravate their suicidality (e.g. a parent who is persistently hostile and dismissive to their child, preoccupied by their own difficulties, or is unresponsive);
  - to allow the family the opportunity to show care and concern, and help to correct the young person's perception of themselves as unworthy, unlovable, 'in trouble' with the parent(s) or deserving of punishment.
- Contact child and adolescent psychiatric services for consultation or to discuss appropriate and timely follow-up.
- Ensure discharge arrangements are safe: to the care of a responsible adult if possible, or consider the need for admission in the interests of the patient's safety.

Because self-harm is the problem you will encounter most frequently, and about which you will be required to know in more detail, there is a chapter devoted to this subject (see Chapter 5).

Psychosis

Acute psychosis in children and adolescents can have organic or functional causes. It is essential to rule out organic causes and not to presume at the onset that the cause is functional. The term psychosis implies that the person has lost the capacity, at least in some areas of functioning, to discriminate internal/mental activity and experience from objective reality (what is real to everyone else). Symptoms include:

- disordered thoughts and incoherent speech;
- hallucinations (e.g. hearing voices that others cannot hear, seeing things others cannot see);
- delusions (fixed, false unshakeable beliefs), including delusions of reference (e.g. a conviction that there are hidden messages in the words of a song or the pronouncements on television programmes, which are meant for the patient specifically); paranoid delusions (e.g. that MI5 are keeping the patient under surveillance); grandiose delusions (e.g. believing oneself to be Christ, a pop star or a friend of famous people, or to have special powers); depressive delusions (e.g. the patient believing that they are guilty of some terrible sin or crime for which they must be punished);
- a sense of external control of or interference with thinking (in schizophreniform psychoses);
- aggression (often based on fear);
- bizarre, manneristic, incongruent, inappropriate and unpredictable behaviour (often accompanied by agitation, fear and high arousal, or alternatively profound withdrawal);
- in the case of mania (or hypomania), relentless overactivity with pressured speech and elated mood (sometimes alternating with fractiousness).

In children and adolescents, the most common cause of acute psychosis is drug misuse, for example the use of amphetamines, cannabis (especially 'skunk'), ecstasy, khat and cocaine. Acute drug intoxication may precipitate acute psychosis that lasts a short time, but it may also precipitate an enduring psychosis to which the young person may already have been vulnerable. Prescribed drugs, especially steroids, can cause psychosis. Other organic causes include brain tumour, head injury, encephalitis and hepatic failure, among others. In some ethnic groups, brief reactive psychotic episodes in the face of severe stress are sometimes seen.

Children and adolescents with severe PTSD, especially the chronic and complex type related to early abuse, may have psychotic-like experiences, including 'flashbacks' and pseudo-hallucinations accompanied by hyperarousal and/or dissociation and derealisation. Dissociation, the disconnection of emotions from thoughts and actions, may be evident as vagueness or even confusion. Derealisation may produce an incongruous indifference, a 'this isn't happening to me' state of mind or even, in extreme cases, out-of-body experiences.

Bipolar disorder (manic depression) and schizophrenia are the main categories of functional psychosis. Bipolar disorder is a disorder of mood, and the person may become psychotic with mood congruent delusions; for example, in a person who is psychotically depressed, nihilistic, negative delusions, and in a person with mania, grandiose delusions together with disinhibition and overactivity. Schizophreniform psychoses affect many areas of the young person's thinking, perception and personality, and usually present gradually over time during adolescence but may present suddenly, especially when precipitated by drug misuse. The clinical picture in adolescents is often a mixed picture with some mood disturbance in addition to the psychotic symptoms.

Management

Keeping the patient and staff safe

- See the child/adolescent in a safe, quiet environment.
- Use calm, non-threatening voice and gestures.
- Remember many people with psychosis are frightened and agitated.
- Do not do anything too quickly or unpredictably unless you need to.
- Explain procedures.
- Allow the young person to express any fears or anxieties.
- Calm and sympathetic supervision by a nurse may be prudent and clinically useful.

Assessment

- Consider organic causes first.
- Check vital signs, including pulse, temperature and blood pressure.
- Always obtain a urine specimen for toxicology if possible before giving medication.
- Do a physical and neurological examination if possible (if the patient is not so agitated that this will be too intrusive and provocative).
- Consider blood tests.
- Be aware of the possibility of dehydration.
- Refer urgently for psychiatric opinion once physical investigations are completed.
- Assess mental state and write down what the patient is saying and doing.
- Obtain as much history as possible from accompanying adults.

Restraint

- Restraint may be necessary if the patient becomes violent (see Chapter 6, pp. 77–79).
- Be aware of legal issues regarding restraint against will and document clearly reasons for using common law.
- Call other staff members and police, if necessary, to keep the situation safe.

Sedation

- Sedation may be required as a last resort (see Chapter 6, pp. 79–85).
- Sedation in an acute presentation is to treat agitation – benzodiazepines are the first choice, especially if the diagnosis is unclear. Offer oral medication prior to considering intramuscular administration. This could also be used prudently as a way of de-escalating a situation, potentially avoiding restraint and the use of intramuscular medication.
- Monitor mental state and level of consciousness and vital signs.

Other issues

In-patient psychiatric management may be required. This may involve use of the Mental Health Act (see Chapter 7). However, child and adolescent psychiatric services have very little access to in-patient beds and, although far from ideal, the young person may remain in the emergency department while future management is determined. Close working and cooperation between the emergency department staff and the psychiatric services is essential. Out of hours, the child and adolescent specialty registrar/ consultant must be contacted.

Anxiety

Experiencing anxiety is normal. However, experiencing severe anxiety is unpleasant and not usually useful, and indeed may impede a young person's ability to plan appropriate responses, take in new information or carry out complex activities, impeding development. Having general anxiety and developing specific fears are among the common emotional problems occurring in childhood.

In the pre-school period (under the age of 5 years), about 9% of children may have up to six fears, three of which may be more marked (and usually situation-specific or transient). Most common fears in children under 5 years would be fears of the dark, thunder, animals and insects. By age 8, only 2% are affected, and this prevalence seems to persist through until the age of 14. In adolescence, specific fearfulness is less common and when it occurs is likely to focus on social situations or take the form of school refusal.

Physical complaints as a result of recurring fears about health – the somatoform disorders – are not anxiety disorders as such, but are associated with high levels of anxiety.

Classification of anxiety disorders

Panic disorder

Children and adolescents experience recurrent and unexpected panic attacks that are followed by worrying about having another attack.

Claustrophobia

This may manifest not only as a fear of enclosed spaces, but also as adolescents or children being concerned about being in a situation from which it would be hard to escape. The anxiety may lead to avoidance of certain situations.

Agoraphobia

This is a fear of open spaces, and leads to fear of going out. It mainly applies to adolescents – younger children tend to present with separation anxiety, which is related – and may be confused with social anxiety/phobia or school refusal.

Social phobia

Adolescents are anxious about being scrutinised or assessed by others in case they do something humiliating.

Specific phobia

Adolescents may have a persistent and irrational fear of a particular object – the fear leads to avoidance of some objects or situations.

Generalised anxiety disorder

This involves worry about a number of different areas of their life to a degree that is excessive and persistent.

Obsessive–compulsive disorder

Experience of unpleasant and intrusive thoughts that are difficult to resist or control; the obsessional thoughts can lead to uncontrollable excessive ritualised behaviours, performed to counteract the thought or prevent the feared/catastrophic event from happening.

Disorders with a specific stressor

Acute stress reaction

In response to a traumatic event, the adolescent or child may present with disorientation, anxiety, amnesia, agitation and withdrawal. They may have all the symptoms of PTSD, but for a brief time only. In the context of the emergency department, acute stress reactions are common after road traffic accidents, traumatic injury and in response to witnessing violence, injury and destruction.

Post-traumatic stress disorder

Adolescents and children may have persistent, intrusive, affectively-charged memories of a previous traumatic event, and may experience generalised hyperarousal, nightmares, flashbacks and avoidance of triggers that may cause them to relive the traumatic event.

Adjustment disorder

Short-lived emotional distress following a significant life change or stressor.

Presentation of anxiety disorders

Hyperventilation

One of the presentations of anxiety to the emergency department is due to the effects of hyperventilation which can accompany anxiety. This may not be obvious to the clinician in casualty. It is possible to have been slightly over-breathing for a long period of time, which perpetuates the state of anxiety. Chronic hyperventilation will produce a marked drop in carbon dioxide and metabolic alkalosis, which may remain subclinical until an episode of acute anxiety leads to exaggerated hyperventilation, the body cannot cope with further decreases in carbon dioxide and acute symptoms are triggered. An adolescent with hyperventilation may present with any constellation of the following symptoms:

- in the brain:
    - dizziness
    - light-headedness
    - confusion
    - breathlessness
    - blurred vision
    - feelings of unreality
- in the body:
    - an increase in heart rate
    - numbness and tingling in the hands and feet
    - cold clammy hands
    - stiffness in the muscles
    - muscle twitching or cramps
    - irregular heartbeats.

Management

The remedy for hyperventilation is re-breathing from cupped hands or from a (small) paper bag, but the importance of reassurance and psychoeducation about the nature and causation of the symptoms cannot be underestimated.

Panic attacks

Presentation to the emergency department may be because of the following symptoms, which are extremely distressing to the young person:

- shortness of breath
- dizziness, tightness or pain in the chest
- faintness
- trembling or shaking
- feelings of unreality
- dry mouth
- muscle tension
- difficulty gathering thought or speaking
- pounding heart

- tingling fingers of feet
- a chocking or smothering feeling
- sweating
- hot or cold flushes
- urge to flee
- nausea or 'butterflies in the stomach'
- blurred vision
- fears of dying, losing control or going mad.

Management

Initially, medical assessment is required to determine whether organic or physical factors underlie the anxiety symptoms. Once these have been excluded, further assessment can focus on identifying the specific nature of the anxiety disorder (pp. 37–38).

When panic attacks occur without any obvious explanation, young people can misinterpret these symptoms as indicating a serious physical or mental problem. These attributions become threatening and can trigger or exaggerate the anxiety response. Depression commonly underlies and exaggerates anxiety in teenagers, and this should always be considered in the assessment.

Management of the acute episode starts with the management of hyperventilation – re-breathing, reassurance and explanation (p. 39).

Understanding the child's or adolescent's anxiety and dealing with this calmly and sympathetically ('containing' the anxiety) will go a long way to relieving the anxiety in many cases.

Managing the parent's/carer's anxiety is essential, so that their anxiety does not aggravate the child's or adolescent's anxiety – the less mature the child, the more they will take reference from the parent's anxiety.

In the adolescent unresponsive to other interventions, benzodiazepines may need to be considered (1 mg of lorazepam is commonly used).

If the panic attacks are recurrent, a referral for specialist help will be needed to provide the non-acute management of the panic attacks, which would normally include psychoeducation, relaxation training and cognitive–behavioural therapy (CBT). In severe, unremitting cases, medication (fluoxetine, buspirone and/or beta-blockers) might be indicated.

Generalised anxiety disorder

The predominant presentation to an emergency department would be one of persistent generalised and excessive feelings of anxiety, which could include:

- nervousness or restlessness
- trembling
- trouble falling or staying asleep
- sweating
- poor concentration

- palpitations
- frequent micturition
- muscular tension
- fatigue
- irritable mood
- light-headedness
- hyper-vigilance
- shortness of breath
- depressed mood.

Routine medical assessment will exclude organic or physical disease. (The medical assessor should be aware that the young patient is of course more likely to present for treatment for the specific symptom, rather than the underlying generalised anxiety disorder.)

A calm and patient assessment will be therapeutic in its own right. As with the management of panic attacks, reassurance and explanation, and the containment of parental anxiety will often be sufficient to interrupt the crisis. The use of sedative medication for generalised anxiety is not encouraged.

Generalised anxiety is not usually managed further in the acute services, but a referral to specialist CAMHS for ongoing work as an out-patient is required. This will include further, more detailed assessment of the underlying psychodynamic, family and social-systemic factors, education about the disorder, strategies for controlling anxiety and reducing the stressors, and perhaps psychodynamic counselling and/or family therapy.

Obsessive–compulsive disorder

This often develops during childhood and early adolescence. There could be presentation to an emergency department, particularly when obsessional thoughts are mistaken for delusions. Children and adolescents may present with:

- distress related to unpleasant recurring thoughts and images;
- overwhelming urges to perform repeatedly specific behaviours (compulsions) interfering with daily life, and intense frustration or fear if prohibited from carrying out these rituals;
- depression;
- anxiety.

Obsessional thoughts are usually concerned with contamination, harm to self or others, blasphemy, violence, sex or other distressing topics. The thoughts are recognised as coming from the individual's own mind, and can involve 'seeing' (intensely, but clearly in the mind's eye) whole scenes or images.

Once the diagnosis is confirmed, management includes education about the nature of their difficulties and referral on to a specialist CAMHS team for treatment. Specialist treatment would usually start with CBT and family counselling, but might include the use of medication (selective serotonin reuptake inhibitors (SSRIs) such as fluoxetine or sertraline) as an adjunct.

Acute stress reactions and PTSD

The core symptoms cluster into three components: hyperarousal, intrusive mental phenomena and avoidance phenomena (Box 4.1).

These are accompanied by intense affect (especially fear) and arousal. They may occur spontaneously (and classically when the child is drifting into sleep or reverie), or may be provoked by specific associative memory cues, which may be external (e.g. cars of a certain colour after an road traffic accident) or internal (e.g. normal feelings of sexual arousal in the aftermath of a sexual assault). These may occur with all the attendant sensory components as if in real time – so-called flashbacks.The child/adolescent may also experience dreams (nightmares), which are recapitulations of the traumatic event.

Management

Acute stress reactions and PTSD in the emergency department are treated as per acute anxiety. Further psychological intervention may be undertaken by more experienced practitioners. Interventions will include the following.

- Psychoeducation about the symptoms of acute stress reactions (that these are normal responses to abnormal experiences, and that in most cases these symptoms are self-limiting) and PTSD.

Box 4.1 Core symptoms of acute stress reactions and PTSD

Hyperarousal
- Restlessness (although in cases in which the avoidant symptoms are strongest, inertness may be a feature)
- Jumpiness (enhanced startle reflex)
- Irritability
- Insomnia
- Night terrors and other Stage 4 sleep phenomena such as sleep walking
- Impaired concentration and attention

Intrusive mental phenomena
- Images
- Thoughts
- Memories of the traumatic event

Avoidance phenomena
- Behavioural: avoidance of (potential or actual) memory cues (e.g. avoiding going near traffic or into vehicles after an road traffic accident)
- Affective: becoming over-controlled and emotionally restricted or even numb and dissociated, or in young children, sleepy

---

- Distraction from rumination is usually advised, depending on the nature of the traumatic event.
- Brief counselling to reverse tendencies to 'survivor guilt' and self-blame (powerful predictors of chronicity in PTSD) and to reinforce coping and survival instincts and skills. Where children and adolescent's want to talk about the events, this should be supported by active listening, providing continual interruption to the tendency to internal preoccupation ('trance'), making reference to the traumatic event being in the past and by reconstructing (new) meaning ('making sense') and order ('narrative coherence'). Passively listening to the child 'ventilating' and/or forcing the child to recount the events without active intervention (what some might think of as traditional 'debriefing') are discouraged.
- Family counselling to enhance emotional support without over-compensation. Especially in younger children, the parents' response to the traumatic event is important to evaluate – the younger the child, the more they will take reference from their parents' emotional state; where parents are unable to provide emotional support because of their own traumatised state, consideration should be given to finding alternative temporary carers within the child's familiar family or social network where possible.
- In established, chronic PTSD, depressive symptoms commonly feature and may indicate risk of suicide, especially where PTSD has been long-standing and unrelenting – this should specifically be assessed. (Note: complex PTSD commonly underlies chronic repetitive self-harm and eating disorders.)
- Extreme distress and overarousal may be treated with sedative medication.
- Recurrent nightmares may be curtailed by 'dream rehearsal' – practising recounting the content or theme of the dream in an alert state, with a different, more favourable resolution.
- Established PTSD is not necessarily self-limiting, and should prompt a referral on to specialist CAMHS resources for specific trauma-related psychotherapeutic intervention.
- Occasionally, medication (SSRIs, clonidine) is useful in resistant cases, but should not be prescribed in the emergency department.

Eating disorders

Background

- Anorexia nervosa and bulimia nervosa are relatively more common in adolescence. They are more prevalent in girls but also occur in boys.
- Anorexia nervosa is the third most common chronic illness in adolescent girls after obesity and asthma. The onset is usually post-

puberty but can occur before puberty. Bulimia nervosa is typically seen in older adolescents or in young people who have anorexia and then go on to develop bulimia.

Both anorexia and bulimia have a high morbidity in terms of the young person's physical, social and academic functioning. There can be serious physical and psychiatric complications.

Young people with anorexia often present very late to medical services, having concealed or minimised their problems to their family and friends. On presentation, they may be physically compromised and sometimes in a state of severe starvation.

Presentation

Presentation to the emergency department may be because of physical symptoms including:

- fainting
- weakness
- cold/hypothermia
- collapse
- vomiting
- diarrhoea (laxative misuse).

Presentation may also be due to psychological symptoms including:

- self-harm (the incidents of self-harm in patients with eating disorders is high)
- low mood
- suicidal thoughts
- marked agitation.

Management

- Take a careful history. Remember that the rate of weight loss and/or extremely limited food/water intake may be more worrying signs than actual body weight.
- Do a careful physical examination including:
  - pulse (patients often are bradycardic and may have an arrhythmia);
  - blood pressure (lying and standing – look for postural drop), blood pressure often low;
  - signs of dehydration;
  - temperature – may be extremely hypothermic;
  - cold extremities.
- Vomiting and/or laxative misuse – the young person may have low potassium levels (potentially life threatening). Do blood test if necessary.

- If concerned about physical state (usually prompted by a combination of a body mass index of <16, bradycardia of <60 beats per minute, diastolic blood pressure of <50 mmHg, and hypothermia of <36°C), consider admission to a paediatric ward (or adult medical ward for older adolescents if this is the policy in your hospital). Remember anorexia nervosa can be a life-threatening condition and a patient in an extreme physical state is unlikely to be able to respond to your advice to eat or drink more.
- Self-harm/depression: consider contacting CAMHS urgently or make urgent out-patient referral.
- If the young person is not known already to CAMHS, consider making an urgent out-patient referral (with young person's/family's permission). If permission not given, contact the GP urgently.
- Remember, the young person may not have contacted medical services before and this may be the opportunity to start organising appropriate help.
- Discharge the patient to the care of the responsible adult.

Attention-deficit hyperactivity disorder

Attention-deficit hyperactivity disorder (ADHD) is characterised by inattention, hyperactivity and impulsivity to a degree that is inconsistent with the developmental level of the child and is present in more than one setting. It occurs in approximately 6% of the population.

Some children have a diagnosis of attention-deficit disorder when they have marked problems with inattention and impulsivity but are not overactive.

Core symptoms

Inattention

For example, problems sustaining attention/concentration; difficulty following through instructions and completing tasks; easily distracted; problems organising themselves; makes careless errors.

Overactivity

For example, fidgets excessively; often leaves their seat (e.g. in classroom); runs and climbs and is generally much more active than other children; unduly noisy when playing (compared with other children of the same age); adolescents may be less active, but overtalkative and have feelings of restlessness.

Impulsivity

For example, finds it very diificult to wait their turn or to wait in queues; often blurts out answers before the question has been completed; often interrupts others' conversations; acts on impulse without thinking of consequences of actions.

Of course, many children show these characteristics, but a diagnosis of ADHD/attention-deficit disorder is made when they are present to an unusual degree compared with other children of the same age and developmental level. Children usually become less active and less impulsive as they get older, so a normal level of activity and normal concentration span in a 3-year-old is not the same as the normal level in a 10-year-old.

Additional features

Other features that sometimes present include:

- problems with planning and organisation
- oppositional behaviour
- reckless and dangerous behaviour
- difficulties with peer relationships
- reading problems
- anxiety and sometimes depression
- low self-esteem
- tics
- antisocial behaviour and sometimes involvement with the police.

How these children may present in an emergency

Children with ADHD are most likely to come into contact with the emergency department as a result of an accident: they are more likely than their peers who do not have ADHD to be involved in road traffic accidents (e.g. following impulsive, reckless behaviour when a pedestrian or on a bike) or accidents following other dangerous behaviour.

Some children with ADHD are on medication, most commonly stimulant medication such as methylphenidate or dexamphetamine. Overdose in children with ADHD is unusual but emergency department staff should be aware that medication overdose is dangerous, and that these types of medication also have a 'street value' and can get into the wrong hands. See also *Side-effects of psychotropic medication*, pp. 53–55.

Medically unexplained symptoms

Children and adolescents commonly present to primary care, secondary care and in schools with physical symptoms that have no specific organic cause, or where the severity of the physical symptoms is much worse than would be expected given the organic problem.

'Medically unexplained symptoms' subsumes psychosomatic difficulties, somatisation, dissociative and conversion disorders. The umbrella term is useful. That it is 'medically unexplained' does not necessarily imply a wholly psychological aetiology for the problem. There is often a strong interplay of physical and psychological factors, for example in some recurrent headaches in adolescence.

Common somatic complaints with a large psychological element in children and adolescents include abdominal pain, headache and limb pains. Back ache with a predominately psychogenic origin is rare in childhood (although more common in adolescence) and should be thoroughly investigated to exclude an organic cause. The somatic complaints are often very distressing to the child/adolescent.

Recurrent abdominal pain occurs in 10–20% of children, most frequently those aged 5–12 years. Other symptoms may be present such as nausea or headaches.

In some cases, there is a clearly identifiable cause (e.g. urinary tract infection) which is more likely if the pain is localised rather than diffuse. It is not uncommon as a presenting symptom in girls who have been sexually abused.

Headache is another common symptom, occurring in adolescence and childhood. A good history and examination is essential to try to differentiate headaches with a clearly organic origin (e.g. infected sinuses, cerebral tumour). Medically unexplained headaches and migraine are uncommon in children under the age of five. Migraine is fairly common in childhood and adolescence. Symptoms of medically unexplained headaches often include a tight feeling around the head and there may be a clear pattern of the headaches occurring, for example, mainly on school days.

Medically unexplained physical symptoms in adolescents are common, especially in girls. They include heart pounding, the feeling of having a lump in the throat, pains in limbs, headaches, fainting, chest pains and dizziness.

Dissociative and conversion disorders occur more often in adolescents than children, particularly in girls. Complaints may include limb weakness (and sometimes inability to walk), visual, speech or hearing disturbance or impairment, unusual movements, pseudoseizures (which may occur in patients who are known to suffer from epilepsy) and unexplained collapses. There may be marked inconsistencies in the symptoms and signs: for example, the young person complains of being unable to weight bear but is clearly able to do so with no problem when not watched directly. Often the person shows relatively little distress about the symptoms.

Management

- If possible, obtain previous notes to look at the medical history, which may show consultations for similar medically unexplained problems.
- It is essential to validate the child's symptoms and not dismiss them out of hand or suggest that the child is deliberately making them up. Even if it is thought that the symptoms are largely psychogenic, they are very real to the child.
- Be cautious about overinvestigating; there is a fine line to be drawn between taking the problems seriously, ruling out serious organic

- disorder and overinvestigation, which may result in perpetuating the physical symptoms.
- Physical investigation may be necessary and, if negative, can be reassuring to the young person and family. Repeated and prolonged investigation is often unhelpful and can perpetuate the problem unnecessarily. Consider carefully the need for further investigation.
- Good liaison with the paediatric/adult medical services is essential, especially if the child is previously known to them. Good communication with the child's GP is also essential.
- Admission may be required occasionally, for example if the young person is unable to walk, or is experiencing prolonged or repeated pseudoseizures. Good liaison with the admitting services is essential, including a detailed description of the history obtained and the observations in the emergency department.

Alcohol misuse

Alcohol misuse places a considerable burden on health services and on emergency departments. It is responsible for about 10% of unselected attendances at emergency departments and a higher percentage of presentations with trauma. Alcohol is often consumed with an overdose of tablets or associated with other forms of self-harm. Alcohol misuse is common in adolescents and also sometimes occurs in younger children.

Intoxication

- Young people who present to emergency departments in an intoxicated state can cause major management problems for staff and other patients. The young person may be uncooperative with assessment, or violent towards property, staff or other people.
- There may be concern about the premature discharge of intoxicated patients from the emergency department (at the patient's wish), especially if comorbid physical or mental health problems are suspected.
- Many young people who present with alcohol intoxication have underlying individual, family or social problems that need attention.

Self-harm and alcohol

- Self-harm is often associated with alcohol consumed shortly before or during the episode. In addition, alcohol dependency is associated with an increased risk of suicide. The young person who is intoxicated may not admit to having taken an overdose of tablets. Binge drinking in some young people may be a form of self-harming behaviour in itself.

Mental health assessments are clearly problematic while the young person is intoxicated. If emergency department staff are concerned about their mental state, then arrangements should be made for a mental health assessment to be carried out when the young person is sober but still in hospital – this requires admission, or remaining in the emergency department depending on the local protocols. Even though the mental health professional will not be able to do a proper assessment while the patient is inebriated, they may be able to offer valuable advice on managing the patient and contribute to decision-making, without necessarily assuming clinical responsibility for the patient, who should remain with the emergency department staff until assessment indicates that responsibility should be handed over to the mental health team. Social Services may also be involved.

Alcohol withdrawal syndromes

Severe alcohol withdrawal syndromes in adolescence seem to be uncommon, but because of the trend for young people to begin drinking heavily from an earlier age, withdrawal syndromes may be seen more often in younger children in the future. The features of alcohol withdrawal (in adults) include:

- early withdrawal: symptoms occur up to 12 h after the last drink, and include tremor, sweating, nausea, insomnia and anxiety;
- moderate withdrawal: the signs are more marked, and may include transient auditory hallucinations in clear consciousness;
- withdrawal fits: these can occur from 12 to 48 h after the last drink. They are more likely if there is a previous history of withdrawal fits or epilepsy;
- severe withdrawal/delirium tremens: this usually develops 72 h after the last drink, and carries an increased mortality and morbidity. Clinical features include tremor, agitation, restlessness, fearfulness, hallucinations, autonomic disturbances, sweating, pyrexia and dehydration.

Risk factors for delirium tremens include a severe or prolonged history of alcohol dependency, a past history of delirium tremens and concomitant acute illness.

Management

- If a young person presents with a Glasgow Coma Scale (GCS) score of 14 or below (Teasdale & Jennett, 1974) as a result of alcohol intoxication, then admission is indicated.
- Remember that many young people who are intoxicated have underlying individual, family and social problems that may need addressing.
- Concerning factors may include:
  - drinking alone
  - drinking during the day
  - the younger the child, the greater your concern should be
  - intention when drinking: for example, is the young person drinking socially with friends or drinking alone to get drunk?

- If you think the young person is in immediate danger (from themselves or others), consider admission.
- If you think the young person needs a mental health assessment, then keep them in hospital until sober enough for one to be carried out. Contact CAMHS according to local protocols.
- If you are concerned about the home situation or about the possibility of abuse, contact local Social Services. If you think it urgent, contact the duty social worker (according to local protocol). Follow locally agreed child protection guidelines.
- Remember that an intoxicated young person may also have taken an overdose of tablets or of illegal drugs, but may not volunteer this information.
- Always remember that an intoxicated young person can come to harm accidentally, for example by falling, being involved in a road traffic accident, being involved in a fight, having unprotected sex, and the risk of abuse of someone who is intoxicated. Plan discharge from the emergency department accordingly or consider admission.
- The medical management of severe alcohol withdrawal includes:
  - close observation of vital signs
  - correction of dehydration and electrolyte imbalance
  - treatment of concomitant illness
  - benzodiazepine withdrawal schedule.
- Always discharge the young person under the age of 16 into the care of a responsible adult.

Substance misuse

Many young people try taking drugs and some engage in regular drug misuse.

- Cannabis is the most commonly used drug among 11- to 24-year-olds. It is usually smoked but sometimes baked into food.
- Solvents (e.g. glue, butane gas, aerosols) can be sniffed, sprayed or breathed in from a bag. Solvents make people feel high, cause sleepiness, vomiting and sometimes hallucinations. Solvent inhalation can cause death.
- Ecstasy comes in a variety of tablet shapes and colours. Some people become excitable and euphoric, others extremely anxious and panicky. Ecstasy is more dangerous if the person is dehydrated and can result in collapse and death.
- Amphetamines can be swallowed, sniffed, smoked or injected. People can become very euphoric, irrational and do dangerous things, or may become scared and low in mood, and sometimes hallucinate.
- Lysergic acid diethylamide (LSD) causes hallucinations and an LSD 'trip' can be pleasant or terrifying and can last for several hours. Flashbacks sometimes occur several months later.

- Cocaine can be sniffed or dissolved and injected. Crack cocaine is smoked and has more rapid and intense effects than cocaine powder. Cocaine can cause chest pains and difficulty breathing. Both are highly addictive.
- Heroin is smoked, sniffed or injected. It is highly addictive and can cause fatal respiratory distress.

Reasons for attendance at the emergency department

Patients often present to emergency departments with medical complications associated with their substance misuse. These complications include:

- the direct pharmacological action of the drug itself, for example accidental overdose is a frequent reason for attendance and is the most common cause of death among intravenous opiate users;
- the hazards related to the method and route of drug administration, for example injection sites with abscesses, arterial occlusion, hepatitis;
- the young person's general lifestyle, for example poor social and dietary conditions, self-neglect, exposure to violence;
- some emergency departments are the site of needle exchange schemes.

Other psychosocial difficulties

- Likelihood of poly-drug misuse/dependence.
- Increased risk of psychiatric morbidity (dual diagnosis).
- Increased risk of non-accidental overdose.
- Social difficulties with poor or non-existent accommodation.
- Chaotic peripatetic lifestyle.
- Presenting to services only when in crisis.
- Often the young person is regarded as demanding and difficult, and is unpopular with medical and nursing staff.
- A child may present with intoxication of a drug (e.g. methadone) intended for an adult.

Drug-seeking presentations

Sometimes young people who misuse substances may access emergency departments solely in an attempt to obtain controlled drugs. Some might claim withdrawal and request prescriptions for drugs (e.g. benzodiazepines). Others may claim to have had their prescribed drugs stolen. Often they may present out of hours when it is difficult to confirm their story.

Management

Many substances that are misused (both in intoxication and withdrawal) can give rise to acute psychiatric complications such as stimulant-induced psychosis, panic reactions and delirium. The clinical picture may be complicated by the use of a number of drugs.

- It is probably best to let the drug effects wear off. There may be times when it is necessary to control symptoms by using additional medication.
- General principles involve the patient being nursed, where possible, in quiet, secluded, safe and well-lit surroundings. Give reassurance that the drug effects will wear off in time.
- Explain any procedures in a calm, unhurried manner.
- Monitor hydration and vital signs.
- Obtain a urine specimen for subsequent drug testing.
- Remember that young people who misuse substances have an increased risk of death from suicide, and take seriously any complaints of suicidal thoughts or threats of self-harm.
- Remember young people who misuse substances may already have taken a non-accidental overdose of medication. Take blood samples if suspicious.
- Remember that young people who misuse substances may have comorbid medical and psychological disorders which may require attention.
- The younger the child who has engaged in substance misuse, the greater your concern should be (e.g. seek help for a 10-year-old who has misused solvents).
- If you believe the young person is in immediate danger to themselves or others, consider admission.
- If you are concerned about the home situation or you have concerns about child protection issues, contact Social Services. If urgent, contact the duty social worker. If not urgent, it can wait until the following day. (Follow local protocols.)
- Young people under the age of 16 should only be discharged to the care of a responsible adult.

Factors increasing index of concern in young people who use illicit drugs

Drug taking, especially smoking cannabis, is common in adolescence and is often a group activity. For the majority the risks are limited. Because of this, young people (and professionals) may underestimate the risks of drug taking. However, in the following cases, drug taking may be more risky or indicative of other risks.

- Misuse of drugs such as amphetamines, barbiturates, opiates and cocaine is less common and more serious. Children misusing these drugs are at a much higher risk of developing dependency.
- Individuals who misuse substances have an increased risk of death from suicide. Take seriously any complaints of suicidal thoughts or threats of self-harm.
- High-potency cannabis increases the risk of psychotic disorder.
- The younger the child, the greater the concern (e.g. seek help for a 10-year-old who has misused solvents).

- Where drug taking is a solitary rather than social activity.
- When there are other risk-taking behaviours (e.g. forensic history, alcohol misuse, self-harm, sexual promiscuity).
- Where there is poly-substance misuse.
- The chronicity and frequency of drug taking is an indicator of risk (of dependency and comorbidity).
- Where there are frank signs of dependence.
- In cases where the young person has poor social support and a chaotic social/home background, for example young people who are:
  - looked after by Social Services or were in Local Authority care
  - involved with the criminal justice system;
  - excluded from education and/or have special education needs;
  - homeless or insecurely housed.
- Where there are evident comorbid mental health problems.
- Where there is evidence of significant social, physical and psychological impairment of functioning.
- Young people whose parent(s) and/or family members misuse drugs and alcohol are at greater risk of dependency (and comorbid problems).

Clearly, where the index of concern is heightened, management plans need to be that much more robust. This may affect the decision whether to admit or not.

Side-effects of psychotropic medication

Psychotropic medication can produce side-effects, affecting all bodily systems, which may lead to presentation in the emergency department. These can be grouped according to the class of drug. Children are particularly vulnerable to neurological side-effects because of the effects on the immature nervous system and developing brain. The clinician will, when encountering these effect, have to decide whether to stop the medication or merely reduce the dose, depending on the severity of the symptoms, or whether to treat with an antidote (where available – see below). Psychoeducation is vital – the patient and parent/carer will be relieved to understand the basis of the symptom, and the 'treatability'.

Antipsychotics

- Children, and especially those with intellectual disability, are particularly vulnerable to extrapyramidal side-effects such as dyskinesia, restlessness and stiffness. Acute dystonias are the most common and occur after a few doses – the most common form is the oculogyric crisis. This should be treated with anticholinergic medication such as procyclidine, at adult doses (5 mg orally or intramuscularly immediately) for post-pubertal young people and a half dose or less for younger children.

- Rare, but potentially fatal, is neuroleptic malignant syndrome, which presents with hyperthermia, muscular rigidity, autonomic dysfunction leading to sweating, pallor, tachycardia and unstable blood pressure. This is a medical emergency. Antipsychotic medication must be stopped immediately.
- Reduction in seizure threshold causing onset or worsening of seizures.
- Anticholinergic effects: dry mouth, blurred vision, urinary retention, constipation.
- Photosensitivity causing sunburn. The patient should be given advice about avoiding harsh sunshine.
- Postural hypotension causing faints is common. More rarely, cardiac arrhythmias may occur. Keep the patient prone, elevating legs if necessary. Stop or reduce medication. The prescribing clinician may wish to change to medication with less cardiovascular activity.
- Hypersalivation, especially with clozapine. Treat with atropine-like medication such as Kwells.

Antidepressants

Selective serotonin reuptake inhibitors

- Most common: gastrointestinal side-effects such as nausea, vomiting, diarrhoea, dyspepsia, decreased appetite, abdominal pain and constipation. These usually gradually wear off after a few days.
- Agitation, insomnia, nightmares and headaches are also common.
- Very rare but serious is serotonin syndrome (caused by SSRI-promoted serotonin hypersecretion), presenting with fever, rigors, sore throat, diarrhoea, tachycardia, restlessness, agitation, confusion, tremor and nausea/vomiting. The SSRI must be discontinued immediately.
- Rare: syndrome of inappropriate antidiuretic hormone secretion, which should be suspected in those presenting with hyponatraemia, with drowsiness, confusion and seizures.
- Hypersensitivity rashes are rare but may be a sign of an impending serious systemic reaction. Also occasionally angioedema, urticaria and photosensitivity.
- Withdrawal symptoms resemble symptoms of serotonin syndrome. Treat by re-prescribing a lower dose of SSRI and withdrawing more slowly or by psychoeducation if mild and bearable.

Tricyclic antidepressants

- Potentially fatal in overdose.
- Anticholinergic effects: dry mouth, blurred vision, urinary retention, constipation.
- Uncommon: severe headache, nausea, postural hypotension.
- Rare: tremor.

Anxiolytics

Benzodiazepines

- Sedation, hypotension, paradoxical disinhibition.
- Withdrawal symptoms include agitation and insomnia.

Buspirone

- Agitation, anxiety and restlessness.
- Postural hypotension causing faints.
- Gastrointestinal disturbance: nausea, vomiting and diarrhoea.

Methylphenidate

- Common: sleep disorders, tics (worsening or new onset), agitation.
- Rare: hallucinations, tremor, epistaxis, urticaria, pruritus, chest pain and severe headache.
- Very rare: jaundice, cerebral arteritis, anaemia, thrombocytopaenic purpura, leucopaenia.

Mood stabilisers

Carbamezapine

- Common: allergic rash, nausea and vomiting, diarrhoea/constipation.
- Dose related and reversible: diplopia, ataxia, dizziness.
- Extremely rare: blood dyscrasias, liver damage, cardiac arrhythmias.
- Syndrome of inappropriate antidiuretic hormone.

Sodium valproate

- Common: nausea, vomiting and diarrhoea, and allergic rashes (up to 14 days after starting).
- Rare: liver damage, disturbed platelet function and other blood dyscrasias.

Lamotrigine

- Common: nausea and mild rash.
- Rare: blurred vision, diplopia, ataxia, photosensitivity causing sunburn.
- Very rare: Stevens–Johnson syndrome, bone marrow suppression causing anaemia, bruising and infection.

Lithium

- Fine tremor, nausea, vomiting and diarrhoea, and polydipsia/polyuria are common. Lithium can cause renal failure.
- Hypothyroidism, oedema and skin rashes are rarer.
- Lithium toxicity causes: blurred vision, drowsiness, confusion, slurred speech, polydipsia/polyuria, dizziness and vomiting, ataxia, severe tremor.

Altered conciousness/altered mental status

Altered mental status in a child is defined as the failure to respond to the external environment in a manner appropriate to the child's developmental level, despite verbal and/or physical stimuli. It denotes impairment of awareness and arousal, the two components of consciousness.

Patients with altered mental status require simultaneous stabilisation, diagnosis and treatment to maintain life and prevent irreparable central nervous system damage.

There is a spectrum of mental status alteration that can occur from mild confusion to coma. This corresponds to a range of conditions including disorders in perception and states of decreased awareness.

Irrespective of the cause, altered mental status indicates depression of both cerebral cortices or localised abnormalities of the ascending reticular activating system. Classic causes of cerebral depression include toxic and metabolic states that deprive the brain of normal substrates. Any abrupt interruption or selective destruction of the reticular activating system can lead to altered mental status.

There are three main pathological categories into which the causes of altered mental status fall: supratentorial mass lesions, subtentorial mass lesions and metabolic encephalopathy. There are features in the history and examination of the patient that are suggestive of cause. For example, supratentorial lesions often cause focal motor abnormalities from compression; subtentorial lesions lead to reticular activating system dysfunction and rapid loss of consciousness; metabolic encephalopathy usually causes depressed consciousness before depressed motor signs with early respiratory involvement.

Diagnosis depends on a comprehensive history including prodromal events, exposure to toxins and the likelihood of abuse.

Examination must include the Glasgow Coma Scale (GCS) with appropriate paediatric modification and an understanding that to be useful it must be reassessed regularly (Table 4.1).

The scale comprises three tests: eye, verbal and motor responses. The three values separately as well as their sum are considered. The lowest possible score (the sum) is 3 (deep coma or death), and the highest is 15 (fully awake person).

Generally, comas are classified as:

- severe, with GCS score ≤8
- moderate, with GCS score 9–12
- minor, with GCS score ≥13.

For children under 5 years, the verbal response criteria are adjusted as shown in Table 4.2.

The differential diagnosis is wide and the mnemonic 'AEIOU TIPS' remains commonly taught: A, alcohol, acid-based and metabolic disorders, arrhythmias and other cardiogenic causes; E, encephalopathy,

Table 4.1 Glasgow Coma Scale

	1	2	3	4	5	6
Eyes	Does not open eyes	Opens eyes in response to painful stimuli	Opens eyes in response to voice	Opens eyes spontaneously	N/A	N/A
Verbal	Makes no sounds	Incomprehensible sounds	Utters inappropriate words	Confused, disoriented	Oriented, converses normally	N/A
Motor	Makes no movements	Extension to painful stimuli	Abnormal flexion to painful stimuli	Flexion/ withdrawal to painful stimuli	Localises painful stimuli	Obeys commands

Reproduced with permission from Teasdale & Jennett (1974).

endocrinopathy; I, insulin, intussusception; O, opiates; U, uraemia; T, trauma, thermal, tumour; I, infection, intracerebral vascular disorders; P, poisoning, psychogenic; S, seizure.

With or without a cause being known, the patient is resuscitated, stabilised and has reversible causes reversed (e.g. naloxone is given for opiate toxicity). The involvement of critical care teams is crucial at the outset if required and the care of family and friends of the patient must not be overlooked.

Abuse and neglect

Child abuse or neglect may present to hospital in a number of different ways, some of which may appear to result from mental health problems. Early identification and careful and sensitive handling are essential (see Chapter 8).

Table 4.2 Adjusted Glasgow Coma Scale criteria for children under 5 years

Score	2 to 5 years	0 to 23 months
5	Appropriate words or phrases	Smiles or coos appropriately
4	Inappropriate words	Cries and consolable
3	Persistent cries and/or screams	Persistent inappropriate crying and/or screaming
2	Grunts	Grunts or is agitated or restless
1	No response	No response

Adapted from Reilly et al (1988).

Distressed children and adolescents

Distress is a normal emotional response to pain, discomfort or fear. It is not a sign of mental illness. Most distress on the part of children, adolescents and their families in the emergency department is not in the province of CAMHS.

Distress as a concomitant of physical illness/trauma

The physician/paediatrician is responsible for the holistic care of the patient. This includes helping the patient (and their family) cope with the distress of pain, discomfort, uncertainty and the fear of the unknown, of procedures and of hospitalisation. The CAMHS professional may have a role later on in the process if the child's or adolescent's responses seem exaggerated, but hardly ever have a role in these cases in the emergency department. Occasionally, the CAMHS professional on call may be consulted about appropriate sedation when nothing else has worked to calm the patient down. Usually, however, a calm, patient, sympathetic attitude to the young patient and their carers, and appropriate pain relief will produce the required effect. Paediatric junior doctors should be taught and have supervision regarding these aspects of care.

Distress as a consequence of social adversity

Sometimes young people present to the emergency department in a distressed state because they do not have the means to look after themselves and life has become too stressful to go on living where they have been living, whether at home, in a hostel or on the streets. This is a matter for Social Services, although in some areas it is the voluntary sector that provides the most useful resources in an emergency. It is not a matter for CAMHS, unless the young person has significant comorbid mental health problems.

Intellectual disability

Approximately 3% of the general population have an intellectual disability defined as an IQ <70. At least 1 in 100 of the general population has an intellectual disability to such a degree that they will need highly specialised health services at some point in their childhood.

The full range of psychiatric disorders is seen in young people with intellectual disabilities, although their presentations may not be typical, for example because of communication problems or aggression as a result of physical pain.

A number of other disabilities and disorders frequently occur in association with intellectual disability, such as cerebral palsy, epilepsy, sensory impairments, speech disorders or autism-spectrum disorders.

Communication

Hearing and speech difficulties are more common and may therefore hinder communication. Young people with an autism-spectrum disorder may have specific communication problems. Some people with learning disabilities use alternative communication systems (e.g. picture cards). Distress may be communicated in other ways, such as aggressive behaviour, self-injurious behaviour and withdrawal.

Common presentations

These include physical injuries (e.g. falls, accidental ingestion of unwanted substances); and medical illnesses (e.g. epileptic seizures, marked constipation). Physical illness may present with a change of behaviour, for example aggression may indicate pain. Psychiatric problems present in a number of ways.

- Change in behaviour, for example more withdrawn (people with intellectual disabilities may become depressed, sometimes severely, but may not be able to communicate feelings of distress or despair).
- Aggression is frequently the presenting symptom for a range of mental health problems as well as physical problems.
- Self-injurious behaviour (e.g. marked head banging, self-biting) may indicate, for example, depression or psychological distress.
- Behavioural disturbance such as an increase in activity or general irritability (occasionally may be the result of changes in medication).
- Self-harm.
- Alcohol misuse is common in young people with mild intellectual disabilities but may indicate an underlying problem such as depression and/or social problems, rather than being the manifestation of the learning disability only.
- Child abuse, including neglect, emotional, physical and sexual abuse. Children and adolescents with intellectual disabilities are at greater risk of all forms of abuse and, of course, may not be able to communicate what has happened to them.
- Serious mental illnesses (e.g. psychosis) occur in young people with intellectual disabilities, but diagnosis can be problematic because of communication or of unusual presentations.

Management

- Use simple language when taking the history and when explaining investigations and treatment. Don't over-elaborate.
- Remember to treat the person with appropriate respect and explain what you are going to do.
- Don't do things suddenly and unexpectedly. Use as low a stimulation environment as possible.

- Use the parents/carers if at all possible to assist in giving the history.
- Remember to ask about changes in behaviour as well as physical symptomatology.
- Use the parents/carers to assist in communication with the young person.
- Assess for physical illness even if that is not the obvious problem at first sight.
- Take time.
- Maintain a high index of suspicion for the possibility of abuse. Contact the local Social Services department (or follow local protocols) if at all in doubt.
- Contact the local CAMHS if you have concerns about the young person's mental health.
- Remember consent issues – having an intellectual difficulty does not in and of itself render the young person 'incapacitous' (see Chapter 7).

Think carefully about appropriate discharge and follow-up. Is there someone accompanying the person on discharge? If not, should there be? Communicate adequately with the young person's GP and any other professionals as appropriate.

Autism-spectrum disorders

Autism-spectrum disorder is an umbrella term used to describe disorders such as autism, Asperger syndrome, atypical autism and other pervasive developmental disorders.

Core problems

Social interaction

For example:

- poor use of interpersonal social cues such as facial expression, eye contact;
- lack of awareness or an unusual response to other people's feelings and, sometimes, to their own;
- difficulty developing relationships with other children, especially when young;
- behaviour can be socially inappropriate with little understanding of social rules.

Communication (both verbal and non-verbal)

For example:

- these children often have delayed speech development and sometimes do not develop the use of speech;

- unusual speech patterns with a lot of repetitive speech, the use of stereotyped and copied phrases and unusual intonation;
- they may not use speech much in a communicative, sociable way and may not communicate even their wishes very readily, but may talk at length about thier own particular interests. Conversation can be very one sided;
- they may have limited understanding of speech. Children with Asperger syndrome often have a very good vocabulary but their understanding of speech can be literal with poor understanding of double meanings of words and idioms.
- non-verbal communication, for example use of gestures, may be poorly developed;
- play tends to be less spontaneous with limited varied imagination.

Resticted, repetitive interests and behaviour

For example:

- preoccupation with certain interests such as street numbers, carwashes, names of footballers. They can develop unusual fascinations (e.g. with plugs, street signs);
- repetitive patterns of behaviour such as repeatedly spinning wheels, lining up objects, rituals, and unusual sensory interests such as smelling things, feeling textures;
- problems with changes in their routine or changes around them;
- problems in coping with the unexpected;
- motor mannerisms such as hand flapping, repetitive rocking.

There is enormous variation among children on the autism spectrum. Some children have learning difficulties which can be severe. Others have normal or above normal intelligence. The amount of language varies: some have no or very little language, others become very talkative but conversation can be one sided. Children with autism, like all children, change and develop as they grow older and typically become more sociable with age. Temperament varies greatly. Some children on the autism spectrum are placid and easy going, others are prone to temper tantrums and aggressive behaviour.

Emergency presentations

Children with autism-spectrum disorder may have any of the psychiatric or emotional problems described earlier in this chapter, and the presentation may depend on the specific disorder rather than on the autism as such. You may be called upon to assess medically a child with autism-spectrum disorder, and the emotional, behavioural and relational aspects of the autism may confuse or impede your evaluation. Management of the more common presentations is described below.

Management

- Children who have both an autism-spectrum disorder and an intellectual disability: see *Management*, p. 59–60.
- Anxiety: many young people with an autism-spectrum disorder are highly anxious. Anxiety may be exacerbated by different stimuli, for example loud noises, too many people, a change of surroundings, people coming too close or the unexpected happening.
    - If possible ask an accompanying adult the best way to approach the young person.
    - Try to avoid doing things suddenly and unexpectedly.
    - Keep explanations short and simple. Prolonged and elaborate explanation can be counterproductive.
- Aggressive behaviour: aggressive behaviour in children with autism can be caused by anxiety. Use parents /carers if possible to help reduce anxiety and aggression.
- Communication: some children with autism have very poorly developed speech and understanding of speech (see *Communication*, p. 59). Others have a good vocabulary but may not volunteer information readily and may take time to process/understand what is being said to them. Don't over-elaborate. Try to use parents/carers to assist in communication.
- Pain threshold and response to injury: some young people with an autism-spectrum disorder have a high pain threshold and may appear relatively indifferent to injury and pain. Examine the child carefully rather than relying on their response, for example when there is a suspected fracture. Some children may panic and have an unusually frightened response to the sight of a small amount of blood.
- Depression and self-harm: children with autism have an increased risk of depression, but, even if they are articulate, they may find it difficult to communicate their feelings and emotions (e.g. feelings of distress, low mood and suicidal thoughts). Follow the local guidelines for admission following any self-harm (see Chapter 5). Contact the local CAMHS team if concerned.
- Abuse: children with an autism-spectrum disorder are vulnerable to being abused and, again, may not be able to communicate this or, in some cases, understand what is happening to them. Maintain a high level of suspicion and contact the local Social Services department if at all in doubt.

Self-harm: issues, assessment and interventions

Tony Kaplan*

Because this is by far the most common mental health problem you will encounter in the emergency department, it has been given its own chapter. This should be read in conjunction with Chapter 3 and Chapter 4, *Depression and self-harm*, pp. 33–34.

Definition

Self-harm is 'intentional self-poisoning or injury, irrespective of the apparent purpose of the act' (National Institute for Health and Clinical Excellence, 2004).

Prevalence

Self-harm is a common problem – each year 25 000 young people under the age of 18 will present to emergency departments in England and Wales having harmed themselves (Fox & Hawton, 2004). (The true figure for the incidents of self-harm in the community is probably eight times as high.)

The most common method of self-harm is self-poisoning (90%), mainly with paracetamol (although increasingly with other analgesics and antidepressants) and about 7% of young people who self-harm present with self-mutilation having cut themselves (Fox & Hawton, 2004).

Self-harm in the under-12-year-old age group is rare; the incidence in adolescents increases markedly from 15 years.

Self-harm is more common in girls than boys by a ratio of 4:1, but completed suicide is more common in boys. Although completed suicide in this age group is relatively rare, it is one of the more common causes of death in this age group.

*With special thanks to Quentin Spender for his contribution (see p. vii).

Risk factors

The main vulnerability factors linked to non-fatal self-harm are specific mental health problems (especially major (clinical) depression) and family problems. Other common risk factors include:

- poverty
- social deprivation or alienation (e.g. new immigrants)
- bullying
- rural isolation
- child abuse (emotional, physical and sexual) and neglect
- a lack of alternative coping strategies or support.

Most episodes of self-harm are unplanned (80%), with the usual precipitant being some experience of rejection – an argument with parents, the break-up of a relationship, exclusion from a peer group. Anger through frustration is often the more accessible, pronounced or obvious affective state of the young person at the time of self-harm, although sadness and demoralisation are often just below the surface, and evident in depressive cognition (thinking patterns). Most young people do not end up with a diagnosis of severe or enduring mental illness. Of those that do, depression is the most common diagnosis, especially in the most severe cases. A sizeable minority have a conduct disorder.

Repetition

About 10% of young people will repeat self-harming themselves. The rate of repetition tends to depend on:

- personality factors (especially impulsivity, hostility and explosive anger, and emerging borderline personality disorder/disorganised attachment);
- circumstances (the persistence or recurrence of the risk factors and stresses above);
- the presence of mental health problems (especially depression, but also substance misuse).

Risk factors for completed suicide include:

- male gender
- older age
- sustained high suicidal intent, with a high and persistent degree of hopelessness (indicating very depressed mood and/or coping skills deficits)
- giving an unclear or fatalistic reason for the self-harm
- having previous episodes of self-harm
- psychosis
- depression

- substance and alcohol misuse (especially a combination of both)
- chronic physical illness
- access to the means of a sudden/violent death (especially guns).

Motives for self-harm are often complex. Relatively few young people who self-harm have an explicit and sustained 'death wish'. Some, especially those who cut themselves repeatedly and superficially, or who take a 'low-risk' overdose (see below) will have no explicit wish to die. Many of those who take an overdose are transiently or intermittently suicidal only, with a competing fear of death and a wish to survive ultimately. Some are fatalistic about survival.

Motives for self-harm include:

- self-punishment (to relieve feelings of guilt or low self-worth in depression);
- an attempt to elicit sympathy or forgiveness, and to pre-empt rebuke, prior to a disclosure of abuse or wrong doing;
- an escape from distress, especially where other avoidant strategies have failed, for example in school phobia, victimisation or anorexia nervosa;
- a 'manipulation' to change aspects of relationships or others' expectations by making them feel guilty or fearful (in some cases where more ordinary ways of achieving these ends have failed);
- a 'cry for help' – a communication of distress especially in situations of motivational conflict, where the young person wants to elicit care from the person they are also angry with, or frightened of, or expecting rejection or rebuke from, or wishing to protect from emotional overload (e.g. a young girl who has been defying her parents, who then needs their support when she is in difficulty and her friends desert her; or a young girl who has always subjugated her emotional needs so as not to bother her chronically ill mother, who then needs her mother's emotional support when she is bullied and ostracised by peers at school);
- sometimes an explicit an identification with people or characters in the media;
- sometimes, in cases of traumatic bereavement, a fantasy of reunion with the deceased.

However, motives other than actual suicide should not be minimised but should be explored and understood, and attempts should be made to resolve conflicts, reduce distress and help the young person achieve more adaptive coping methods. Of course all of this may not be possible in the emergency department, but should inform the attitude of the practitioner and referrals on to more experienced interventionists or decisions to admit to achieve these aims. The possibility of abuse, deliberate (direct) or non-deliberate (by neglect or exposure to abusive environments), should always be considered where young people present with self-harm.

In most cases where the young person has had an explicit wish to die, the wish to be dead is transient. The persistence of this wish, its evidence in the planning and method of the attempted suicide, and the persistence of this wish after the suicidal act, are probably the best indicators of continuing risk of fatal self-harm. This is especially the case when this persistent wish to die is predicated on a sense of hopelessness and futility, and where there are supporting beliefs, for example that others would be better off without them and that loved ones will get over their death (readily).

Self-injury (cutting)

Young people who cut themselves repeatedly, especially when the cutting is superficial, are usually, but not always, motivated differently from young people who wish to die by suicide. Their self-harm is usually a maladaptive coping strategy without any intention to die. Indeed, this form of self-harm may be in the interests of surviving through distress, and diverting the young person from choosing suicide as a way of escaping unbearable tension or distress. This kind of self-harm (which may include other forms of self-injury such as burning or bruising) produces relief (psychological and physiological) from tension, makes emotional pain tangible and gives the young person a sense of control over this intense discomfort, over which they otherwise have no sense of control. In some cases, the self-injury may relieve dissociation (feeling uncomfortably numb or unreal), especially when this is as a result of previous psychological trauma such as sexual abuse or assault.

The Differential Grid for Cutting can be used to assess whether the young person is at low or high risk of self-harm (Table 5.1).

Table 5.1 Differential Grid for Cutting

Relatively low risk	Relatively high risk
Superficial cutting, leading to little bleeding, and scars that heal quickly	Deep cuts, some needing stitching
Nothing to indicate past abuse	A known history of sexual abuse or rape; promiscuous sexual activity; or wildly unpredictable behaviour
No other self-harm	Associated with overdosing
No history of bingeing, vomiting or distorted body image	Associated with an eating disorder
Abstinence, or a sensible attitude to experimentation with drugs and alcohol	Use of drugs or alcohol that is potentially dangerous
Mood changes are transient	Persistent symptoms of depression or anxiety

Reproduced with permission from Spender (2007).

Also consider the young person's family and social relationships and circumstances, and the availability of other, more adaptive coping strategies and help-seeking behaviour.

Management

Triage

Triage should establish the degree of urgency with which the young person should be seen. This should take into account both the young person's degree of distress and agitation, and the need for medical intervention (to reverse the effects of poisons/overdoses (e.g. medicated charcoal after paracetamol overdose) or to stem bleeding). Adolescents who self-harm repeatedly may be more than usually impatient or ambivalent or even hostile to treatment (especially if they have had previous experiences of emergency department staff as dismissive). They may wish to leave the emergency department before they are seen and assessed. Dealing promptly, sympathetically and respectfully with them will reduce the likeliness of this happening.

Attitude of staff to self-harm

Many (young) people who have self-harmed and attended an emergency department say that they are treated with disdain and as deserving of maltreatment because their problem is deemed to be self-inflicted and a waste of the busy health professionals time (e.g. National Institute for Health and Clinical Excellence, 2004; Mental Health Foundation, 2006). Where this is the case, this attitude is misplaced, unfair and in the end counterproductive, and only makes the work of assessment and intervention harder to achieve and take more time. This attitude is strongly discouraged by the Royal College of Psychiatrists' (1998, 2004b) and NICE (2004) guidelines, but is entrenched in some services and professionals, and to reverse it may require training (a greater understanding of these patients' difficulties and motivation will reduce cynicism), consultation from a mental health professional or supervision from senior colleagues.

Psychosocial (mental health) assessment

Comprehensive assessment is a sequential and cumulative task, and should be contributed to by each professional and professional system that the young person comes into contact with, including primary care staff, ambulance services, triage nurses and other emergency department practitioners, as well as paediatricians, adult psychiatrists where they are involved as duty doctors, and specialist CAMHS workers. This comprehensive assessment should include the young person's capacity and ability to consent to treatment, their psychosocial needs, their mental state and the degree of current and future risk. Neither the Royal College of Psychiatrists' (1998, 2004b) nor the NICE (2004) guidelines specifies which professional staff should be involved, but makes it clear that staff who undertake the comprehensive assessment should:

- have been trained to undertake the task;
- have the knowledge, skills and attitudes that are required by the task;
- be able to recognise when they are at the edge of their knowledge, ability or tolerance and be able to request supervision or consultation as appropriate;
- know when and in what circumstances to refer a child or adolescent for further assessment and any necessary action by the consultant child and adolescent psychiatrist or child protection service;
- have an explicit source of supervision or advice available to them, and have explicit access to a consultant child and adolescent psychiatrist for discussion, advice, supervision or consultation as appropriate, and for onward referral of children and adolescents who are thought to require or a more specialised or focused assessment.

The NICE (2004) guidelines state that children and adolescents under 16 years of age should be triaged, assessed and treated by appropriately trained children's nurses and doctors who are experienced in assessing children and adolescents who self-harm, and this should happen wherever possible in a separate children's area of the emergency department. Assessment should include an assessment of the child's family, their social situation and any child protection issues.

Decision to admit

All young people under 16 who have self-harmed should be admitted to hospital to enable a full psychosocial assessment (Royal College of Psychiatrists, 2006a, as well as NICE (2004) guidelines). It is advisable that under 18s are admitted also (and imperative if the risk assessment indicates this), but if this is to be to an adult ward and not to a child or adolescent ward, the balance of advantages and risks may change and the older adolescent's wishes regarding admission need to be given more weight.

Children under the age of 16 years admitted to the paediatric ward should be under the care of a consultant paediatrician, who should, with at least parental consent, arrange an assessment by specialist CAMHS within the next working day.

Decision to discharge

Any decision to discharge a young person from an emergency department without CAMHS assessment following an act of self-harm should be based upon a combined assessment of need and risk. The assessment should be written in the case notes and passed on to the GP and to any relevant mental health services. The Royal College of Psychiatrists, Royal College of Paediatrics and Child Health, and College of Emergency

Medicine urge particular caution with taking this approach in respect of children and adolescents. A paediatrician should always be consulted before staff of an emergency department take action of this kind. The paediatrician may decide to consult CAMHS staff before concluding an opinion. In particular, the decision to discharge a child or adolescent following an act of self-harm should not be based solely upon the presence of low risk of self-harm and the absence of mental illness, because many such people may have a range of other social and personal problems, attention to which may reduce risk in the future. The environment into which they are discharged is of paramount importance – it will be less risky to discharge to a well-supported environment, especially one in which the young person will avail themselves of the help and support offered. Where an appreciable risk still exists at the point of discharge, carers should be made aware of the risks, given guidance on how to judge increasing or diminishing risk (behavioural markers of risk they identify) and urged to be cautious and vigilant, and not to downplay risks. Known risks, for example the ready availability of tablets in the home, should be proactively avoided.

Psychosocial assessment of self-harm

- See *Depression and self-harm*, pp. 33–34, for some general points about conducting an interview with a young person with depression.
- Take a systematic history (sympathetically) of the sequence of events that make up the self-harming episode to inform the risk assessment (see below).
- Elicit the precipitating factor(s): check if there is more than one – it is often the coincidence of more than one stress factor that precipitates the act of self-harm; continue to enquire until the account 'makes sense'/is plausible and coherent.
- Check for current stresses (and whether these are enduring, self-limiting or resolved).
- Explore aspects of the social and family circumstances which may have contributed to their vulnerability, be provocative and exaggerate distress, or conversely provide a degree of protection and comfort, reducing future risk.
- Enquire about previous self-harm episodes/suicide attempts or suicidal ideation, and why these did not result in death (this may make apparent an increasing risk, or conversely elucidate protective or resilience factors or make clear the non-suicidal motivation of the young person).
- Explore possible solutions.
- Make and record accurately a formal risk assessment.
- Make a risk management plan, including admission; consult a CAMHS colleague on call (if they have not been part of the assessment); make a decision as to the level of supervision required to ensure safety,

medication if required to ameliorate agitation and a plan for review; and discharge planning with follow-up or transfer to a tertiary unit.

Suicide risk assessment

There are no established risk assessment tools with a good evidence base when applied to adolescents, although both the PATHOS questionnaire (Kingsbury, 1996) and the Pierce questionnaire (Pierce, 1977) (see *Suicide risk assessment tools*, pp. 74–75) are useful adjuncts to clinical assessment. The risk evaluation is best done by rigorous clinical assessment, balancing the adversity factors (those that increase risk) against the protective factors (those that diminish risk). This is in three domains: evaluating the suicidal act, circumstantial/social factors, and the mental state.

Evaluating the suicidal act

This is best done by tracking the suicidal event chronologically. Examples are given below of the questions you can usefully ask, and what you can infer from the answers.

What happened? What did you do?

The more violent the act that can be expected to kill quickly or even instantly (e.g. using a gun, jumping from a height, hanging (not strangling), cutting deeply enough to open a large vein or artery), the more lethal the intent.

What did you want to happen (from doing that)?

Motives for self-harm are listed on p. 65. Supplementary questions (to elicit inhibiting and coping thoughts) include:

- Have you done anything to try to kill yourself before? If so:
  - how come you didn't die on that occasion?
  - what got in the way?
  - was there anything you remember thinking then that made you change your mind and want to live?
- Have you had suicidal ideas and not acted on them? If so:
  - what put you off then?
  - why did these things not put you off on this occasion?

How long had you thought about it before you did it?

Planning *v*. impulse: the more premeditated the act, the more sinister. For example, someone who saves up enough paracetamol over days and then waits to take them when everyone has left the home is at more risk than someone who takes whatever is to hand minutes after an argument. This is not to say that impulsive self-harm is inherently non-risky – sometimes young impulse-prone people die by suicide almost 'by accident'. The dangerousness may also be related to what they choose to do impulsively to harm themselves – an impulsive overdose may well be reversed somehow and in time, whereas jumping off a bridge impulsively may not be reversible.

Did you do anything to make sure you wouldn't be found in time?

Taking care to plan suicide in such a way as to avoid detection and prevention is, of course, indicative of greater intent to die.

Writing a suicide note is not in itself indicative of lethal intent – it is sometimes written 'for effect', rather than as a last communication; the style, content, and when and how it is found may give some clue to its purpose.

What were you thinking as you were harming yourself/trying to kill yourself?

This is an open-ended question to probe whether there were explicit thoughts of dying and, if so, what the psychological reactions to this were. If there were explicit thoughts of dying:

- were these persistent, transient or intermittent?
- did these thoughts provoke any wishes to be deterred or rescued (especially, the impulse to tell someone, or to call an ambulance)? Did they then act to save themselves, or did they fight against the wish to be rescued?
- having had an explicit wish to die, did they then put this thought out of their mind without taking any action to prevent this from happening (and then, for example, go to sleep)? (This dissociation – disconnecting from feelings – is worrying, especially when trying to develop pre-emptive safety strategies for the future, since the young person may not have a trigger for coping thoughts.)

It is worth checking, in a very young child or an adolescent with moderate or severe intellectual difficulties, whether their ideas about being dead include the idea of death as permanent.

Some young people will have the fantasy of dying in order to join ('in heaven') someone close who has died – this may represent a fantasy (more benign) or a fully-formed belief (more worrying), in some, supported by their religion or culture.

If there were no explicit thoughts of dying, was there instead a fatalistic acceptance of whatever outcome transpired (including death)? (This can also be of concern.)

If you had died (if they confirm they had a death wish), who would have found your body? Who would have been affected?

Having to confront the thought of someone else finding their dead body brings home to the young person the real possibility of their death following a suicidal act and the potential effect on someone else – it is worth checking whether someone they may still feel protective towards (e.g. a younger brother or sister) might have found their dead body. The effect of this question on the parent is often illuminating – if the parent is upset and tearful, this indicates that the protective attachment relationship is functioning, and the young person can count on a caring response from their parent. No response from the parent or sadistic glee in a young person in response to a show of parental concern are both worrying.

The importance of finding out who the young person thinks would have been affected by their death is twofold.

- Some people with depression feel they are a burden to others, and that others will be better off without them (this increases the suicide risk significantly).
- Being aware of how much others care about them and that others would be very upset by their death is something worth amplifying as a thought that may help the young person to resist acting on a suicidal wish in the future.

How was your suicide attempt discovered? Why were you found?

The response to this question will give some indication of the presence of (protective) or absence of (more sinister) an active self-preservation instinct; that is, the overwhelming (although sometimes subconscious) wish to stay alive. For example, it would be worrying if the young person was discovered unconscious or by chance, and especially if they had made attempts to avoid discovery. It is less worrying (from the perspective of assessing lethal intent) if, for example, they took an overdose in front of someone else or called a friend to tell of the overdose (even if they asked their friend not to tell anyone else).

What were your first thoughts when you knew you weren't going to die?

This, and their first thoughts and feelings about being safe, are powerfully predictive – if they were frustrated or disappointed that they hadn't died, this is very worrying.

If they did feel this directly after being 'rescued', but subsequently this changed to relief at being saved and/or regret at having acted on their suicidal impulse, what caused this change in their thinking? What made the switch in their motivation should be highlighted, as it may represent a 'coping' thought or perspective, which, if held in mind at the time, may preserve them/prevent them from acting when they next feel suicidal.

How are you feeling about your circumstances now?

- What has changed?
- What could change?
- What would you need to do to get this change to happen/to enhance desired change?

The circumstances that precipitated the suicide attempt may have changed, perhaps as a result of the attempt – for example, the boyfriend, who had 'dumped' her, may have re-dedicated himself to the relationship; the parents may have rescinded their indefinite grounding for a misdemeanour, etc. These questions elicit hopefulness and engender empowerment (and indicate a positive outcome), or conversely help to identify and address feelings of hopelessness and/or helplessness (which suggest the need for more vigilance).

What difficulties/stresses do you still have to face/deal with (and what will you do about those?)

Be aware that the relief of survival and the sudden rush of family support may bring an initial false optimism – don't discount this, but also explore what still needs to be resolved and what plans there are to deal with it realistically.

What will you do when you next have a suicidal thought?

This helps to identify the coping skills and strategies of the young person, and if convincingly present, help to reduce risk. Coping skills and strategies will often include:

- internal cognitions (e.g. positive self-talk such as 'I am a worthwhile person');
- an awareness of what they want to stay alive for;
- an awareness of why they didn't want to die (e.g. because they wouldn't want to upset their family and friends);
- the capacity to use external support (knowing others cared and wanted to help).

Evaluating the mental state

According to the curricula for training, all junior doctors working in the emergency department should be able to conduct a basic mental state examination (Appendix II). However, if your basic examination leads to heightened concerns, you may wish to have the opinion of a psychiatrist/ psychiatric trainee with more experience in this area.

You will need to pay attention to persistent depressive affect (perhaps indicated by a sad expression, depressive posture, slow speech, withdrawal), and the depressive or psychotic thinking that will usually be evident from your evaluation of the risks as above. It is of course of great concern if the young person has acted on 'command' auditory hallucinations.

Weighing the factors

Risk indicators are then weighed against 'safety' indicators. These will include indicators from your assessment of the patient's circumstances (Box 5.1), your specific risk assessment related to the suicidal act, and the mental state examination. It is usual to err on the side of caution.

Box 5.1 Factors indicating level of risk

Factors increasing immediate risk

- Psychiatric illness: depression (clinical), psychosis, eating disorder
- Unresolved or increasing stress (following the suicide attempt) including:
  - family hostility/rejection
  - continuing victimisation
- Social isolation/reluctance to ask for help
- Alcohol misuse

Factors reducing immediate risk

- Family warm and supportive
- Precipitating stress resolved
- Engaging in therapeutic discussion to produce beneficial change

Suicide risk assessment tools

PATHOS questionnaire

This is a five-question screening instrument to detect high suicidal risk in adolescents who overdose (Kingsbury, 1996). Although there is a lack of good evidence of its reliability, it addresses the five factors that in other studies predict the seriousness of the intention to die, and so it is useful as a quick resume of risk. It should not be used by itself without other assessment, and it does not detect risk of impulsive serious self-harm. The questions are:

- Have you had Problems for longer than 1 month?
- Were you Alone at the time (of the suicide attempt)?
- Did you plan the overdose for longer than Three hours?
- Are you feeling HOpeless about the future?
- Were you feeling Sad for most of the time before the overdose?

Answering affirmatively for two or more of these questions indicates substantial risk.

Pierce Suicide Intent Scale

This is another useful brief checklist (which can be scored) (Table 5.2; Pierce, 1977). Again, this should not be used as the only assessment and should not be administered to the patient as 'boxes to tick'. The therapeutic value to the patient of the clinical assessment is in the clinician's empathy. Furthermore, an 'engaged' patient is more likely to give information honestly.

Table 5.2 Pierce Suicide Intent Scale

Item	Score
Circumstances	
1. Isolation	0 Somebody present 1 Somebody nearby or in contact (e.g. by telephone) 2 No one nearby or in contact
2. Timing	0 Timed so that intervention is probable 1 Timed so that intervention is not likely 2 Timed so that intervention is highly unlikely
3. Precautions against discovery and/or intervention	0 No precautions 1 Passive precautions (e.g. avoiding others but doing nothing to prevent intervention. (Alone in room, door unlocked.) 2 Active precautions (e.g. locked door)
4. Action to gain help during or after the attempt	0 Notified potential helper regarding attempt 1 Contacted but did not specifically notify potential helper regarding the attempt 2 Did not contact or notify potential helper
5. Final acts in anticipation of death	0 None 1 Partial preparation or ideation 2 Definite plans made
6. Suicide note	0 Absence of note 1 Note written but torn up 2 Presence of note
Self-report	
1. Patient's statement of lethality	0 Thought what s/he had done would not kill him/her 1 Unsure whether what s/he had done would kill him/her 2 Believed what s/he had done would kill him/her
2. Stated intent	0 Did not want to die 1 Uncertain or did not care if s/he lived or died 2 Did want to die
3. Premeditation	0 Impulsive, no premeditation 1 Considered act for less than one hour 2 Considered act for less than one day 3 Considered act for more than one day
4. Reaction to the act	0 Patient glad s/he has recovered 1 Patient is uncertain whether s/he is sorry 2 Patient is sorry s/he has recovered
Risk	
1. Predictable outcome in terms	0 Survival certain 1 Death unlikely 2 Death likely or certain
2. Would death have occurred without medical treatment?	0 No 1 Uncertain 2 Yes
Total score[1] =	

1. Low intent, score <4; medium intent, score 4–10; high intent, score >10.

CHAPTER 6

Violence and extreme behaviour

Lois Colling and Eric Taylor*

Circumstances when violence is more likely to occur in the emergency department (see Royal College of Psychiatrists, 2004a) are when the attendees (the young patient as well as to those accompanying the young person, including parents, carers or friends):

- are under the influence of drugs or alcohol;
- have to wait a long time (or where the time they will have to wait is uncertain);
- encounter an uncaring, dismissive or prejudiced attitude on the part of the staff;
- where there is a high degree of anxiety;
- where the patient is in a confused state.

Safeguards include:

- adequate staffing levels (to attend to patients within a reasonable time, and to afford the time to attend to attendees' anxieties respectfully);
- to have a designated member of staff and appropriate mechanisms to inform attendees of the likely wait, reasons for this and progress towards this (e.g. information about facilities that may, for example, reduce discomfort), and for a designated member of staff to have the responsibility of monitoring levels of tension in the emergency department;
- having the availability of appropriately trained hospital security guards and a clear arrangement with the police to attend if necessary;
- identification of patients likely to become violent as an aspect of triage;
- early and prompt attention to violence to prevent or limit escalation;
- a room set aside in which violent patients can be secluded with supervision;
- an alarm system, and protocols for dealing with incidents should the alarm be sounded.

*Eric Taylor acted as Chair of a Paediatric Psychopharmacology Group committee, with special contributions from Gillian Rose and Sean Maskey.

Staff should remember that they have a duty to all the patients in the setting in which they operate – if injured by a violent patient they cannot fulfil their duty to their other patients.

If a violent incident occurs:

- assistance should be summoned immediately – rather too many people to help to ensure safety than too few. Safety of the patient, as well as of the staff and other attendees in the emergency department, is the paramount consideration;
- staff should respond in a calm manner and refrain from angry retaliation;
- a dialogue should be established with the aggressor – the aggressor should feel heard and their underlying feelings (especially fear) addressed.

Following a violent incident or incident in which a violent event was averted, the staff involved should:

- have the need for emotional support validated, normalised and met;
- have supervision if required;
- have the opportunity to debrief – that is, to reflect on the incident to establish what worked well and what did not;
- document the incident (or 'near miss'), with its antecedents and outcomes for learning and audit purposes, and in case of later litigation.

Heads of departments and managers should ensure that:

- all staff are trained in de-escalation techniques;
- all staff are trained in 'breakaway' techniques;
- all departments regularly review safety, early warning and response procedures, and monitor training in dealing with violence;
- all incidents of violence or incidents in which there was a high risk of violence are recorded, reviewed, lessons learned and disseminated, and consequent modifications to procedures implemented – this should be discussed formally in the liaison committee;
- identifying potentially violent situations and defusing them before they escalate is best practice.

Restraint guidelines

For those clinicians involved in the use of restraint (Box 6.1) there must be a clear and regular programme of training, which should cover:

- legal issues
- moral and ethical issues
- the use of clinical holding techniques
- alternative techniques such as distraction and play.

> **Box 6.1 Restraint in children and adolescents**
>
> **Purpose**: Children and adolescents may need to be physically restrained for various procedures because of disruptive behaviour or to prevent injury to themselves or others.
>
> **Planning**: The use of restraint should only occur after careful consideration and rejection of alternative methods, and requires clear indications, safe application and rigid re-assessment guidelines.
>
> **Policy**: In any department or clinical area in which physical restraint procedures may be used, there must be a clear policy available to staff that has been agreed by all those who may be involved with its implementation. This policy should be reviewed at regular intervals and should also be available to patients and their carers.
>
> **Caution**: The use of restraint should never place the child or adolescent at risk of injury or deterioration in their medical condition.

Prior to restraint

- A clear decision must be made by the senior clinician involved in the child or adolescent's care which is discussed with and explained to the other clinicians involved.
- There should then be an explanation to the child or adolescent why a restraint is deemed to be necessary, and what would need to happen for that to be avoided.
- Explanation must then be made to the parent or carers concerning the reasons for restraint.
- All the above should be clearly documented.
- There should be a written order specifying the type of restraint to be used, an estimate of its duration and a time frame for reviewing this (as regularly and frequently as possible).

Restraint

- Restraint must be applied by healthcare professionals who have been trained in the use of restraint with children and adolescents. (Note: techniques used with adults may result in fracture to epiphyses when used in children.)
- The restraint must be correctly applied, with particular regard to skin integrity and neurovascular status.
- The restraint should be accomplished for the purpose for which it is applied, and then should cease.
- Staff should not hold a child in any way that is or could be viewed as indecent, for example exposing the child or adolescent's body unnecessarily, or holding/touching that involves the genital area or breasts. If children have been abused physically or sexually, staff should be

aware that being held even for their own safety might be experienced by the child as a recapitulation of the abuse and be extremely distressing.

- Children's footwear should be removed.
- If restraint occurs in public, other patients, staff and visitors should be asked to leave. Wherever possible the restraint should be carried out in isolation.

Post-restraint

- Debrief the young person (allow them to give critical feedback, and to describe their experience and any resonances this may have had for them).
- Explain again to the young person (and parents) the intended purposes of the restraint and whether the purpose was achieved, and why alternatives were excluded.
- Debrief staff involved (this is often an unpleasant experience for staff, especially those staff who are not required to use physical restraint regularly).
- Complete documentation (including incident reporting if used in an emergency).
- Audit over time.
- Assess training needs and implement training.

Further reading on restraint is listed at the end of this chapter.

Emergency medication and rapid tranquilisation guidelines

Aggressive behaviour includes verbal hostility, threats and intimidation, and overt physical violence. It is the end-point of a variety of events and different mental states. Aggression is a primitive behavioural response that can arise when more complex emotions (e.g. fear, anger, sadness) cannot be articulated or managed internally. Chronic aggression can develop in families where aggression is the preferred communication style or where violence succeeds in resolving conflict. No matter what the cause, the principles of the acute management are the same. The triggers and maintaining factors can be tackled after the patient, staff and other young people are all safe.

The identification of potential aggression is an essential first step. The prevention and de-escalation of aggression is far easier than the direct management of assaultative behaviour.

Assessment

Look out for the following.

- Signs of arousal: pallor, sweatiness, wide-eyed gaze, scanning eye movements, restlessness, shouting.

79

- Disinhibition: history of alcohol or drug intoxication, previous head injury, ADHD and conduct disorder.
- Impaired communication: global learning difficulties, speech and language delay, autism-spectrum disorder.
- Pain: pre-verbal children may be in pain; check ears and teeth.
- Previous aggression: check with carers and hospital records.
- Risk: physical size of patient, possibility of weapons.

Management

Maintain your safety and that of the patient, carer and others.

- If possible remove others from the area.
- Younger patients may be more anxious without carer present.
- Adolescents may be more volatile with carer present.
- Do not be alone with the patient.
- Ensure your colleagues know where you are and bring your panic alarm.
- Use a large room and ensure an escape route for both of you.

Attempt to talk to the young person and to calm them down (Box 6.2).

- Maintain a good distance and go to their eye level (their perception of threat is likely to be heightened).
- Explain what is happening.
- Talk calmly and avoid confrontation.
- Avoid sustaining direct eye contact.
- Ask what they want and meet their needs if possible.

This may contain the situation. Following this, transfer the patient to a more appropriate environment (if available). Some of the later steps will only be necessary if there is actual violence. Obtain and record consent whenever possible.

If physical restraint is required:

- ensure you have sufficient staff to do so safely;
- enlist security guards and porters if necessary;
- do not be afraid to summon the police if necessary;

Box 6.2 Non-drug approaches to calm the severely agitated patient

- Talk to the patient
- Use distractions
- Remove to a low-stimulus area
- Assess the nature of the disturbed mental state
- Exclude causes due to physical illness
- Obtain past and current medication history

- remember that more people will increase the patient's anxiety and potentially their aggression, so act quickly once assembled.

Consider use of medication (rapid tranquillisation).

- Given the small evidence base for the safety and effectiveness of rapid tranquillisation in young people, this should be the final step not the first.
- Ensure you have sufficient people for safe administration of intramuscular medication if oral medication refused.
- Continue to monitor the physical state after rapid tranquillisation.

Oral medication

Children/adolescents with psychosis

In children/adolescents with psychosis, lorazepam (<12 years: 0.5–1 mg, maximum 4 mg/day; >12 years: 0.5–2 mg, maximum 4 mg/day) plus, if needed, either risperidone (0.5–2 mg) or haloperidol (<12 years: 0.5–1 mg, maximum 10 mg/day; >12 years: 1–2 mg, maximum 15 mg/day) together with procyclidine (1.25 mg (<14 years) to 2.5 mg (>14 years)) should be given (Fig. 6.1). Alternatively, give olanzapine (5 mg) as a single-agent treatment in children >12 years.

Non-psychotic/unknown illness

In children/adolescents with a non-psychotic or unknown illness, lorazepam (<12 years: 0.5–1 mg, maximum 4 mg/day; >12 years: 0.5–2 mg, maximum 4 mg/day) or promethazine (<12 years: 5–10 mg; maximum 25 mg/day; >12 years: 10–25 mg; maximum 50 mg/day) (Fig. 6.1).

Caution is advised if using a typical antipsychotic (e.g. haloperidol) for an unknown illness or in an antipsychotic-naïve child/adolescent, as extrapyramidal side-effects may be even more common in children than adults. Because of this, atypical antipsychotics (especially the dispersible forms) are now recommended as the first choice of sedative in this age group. For children under 12/pre-pubertal children, there is no specific dose by weight regime for risperidone – it is advised that the lower end of the dose range is used and only titrated up cautiously if needed. Risperidone quicklets may be more rapidly absorbed and therefore more quickly active than olanzapine velotabs.

When using anticholinergics, attention should be paid to the total anticholinergic effect of all medicines being used. In particular, caution should be taken if using promethazine concurrently with procyclidine due to the increased anticholinergic effects.

If oral medication is repetitively refused, the decision to forcibly medicate (intramuscularly) a child/adolescent will be taken jointly by medical and nursing staff. Once the decision has been made to forcibly medicate, the child/adolescent must be isolated from other children/adolescents on the unit. Nursing and medical staff involved in physically holding and restraining the child/adolescent should be proficient in holding

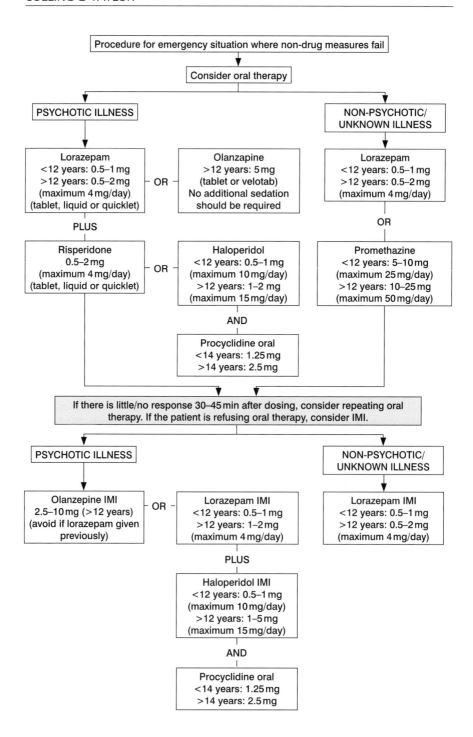

Fig. 6.1 Guidelines for rapid control of younger patients (6–17 years old) who are acutely disturbed. IMI, intramuscular injection. Adapted from Parker & Rose (2004).

and restraint techniques (according to unit-specific policies) and should have adequate immunisation against hepatitis B.

Parenteral medication

The following steps are recommended as parenteral medication regimens for children/adolescents who have not been adequately settled by non-drug measures or oral medication, or who are refusing oral medication.

Children/adolescents with psychosis

In children/adolescents with psychosis, olanzepine intramuscular injection 2.5–10 mg (>12 years only) should be given (Fig. 6.1). Repeat after 30–60 min if necessary up to a maximum dose of 10 mg/day. Olanzapine should not be given with benzodiazepines because of the risk of respiratory depression.

Alternatively, use lorazepam intramuscular injection (<12 years: 0.5–1 mg, maximum 4 mg/day; >12 years: 1–2 mg, maximum 4 mg/ day), repeating after 30 min if necessary, plus (if needed) haloperidol intramuscular injection (<12 years: 0.5–1 mg, maximum 10 mg/day; >12 years: 1–5 mg, maximum 15 mg/day) and procylidine orally (1.25 mg (<14 years) to 2.5 mg (>14 years)) or intramuscularly/intravenously (<10 years, 2–5 mg or >10 years, 5–10 mg). Repeat after 30 min if necessary.

Non-psychotic/unknown illness

In children/adolescents with a non-psychotic or unknown illness, lorazepam intramuscular injection (<12 years: 0.5–1 mg, maximum 4 mg/day; >12 years: 0.5–2 mg, maximum 4 mg/day) should be given (Fig. 6.1) and repeat after 30 min if necessary.

In view of the safety considerations, the intramuscular route is preferable to the instravenous route.

- The maximum *British National Formulary (BNF) for Children* dose of instramuscular lorazepam is 4 mg/day (in adults); at times, doses higher than this may be required. In such circumstances, advice should be sought from senior colleagues.
- Lorazepam should be stored in the fridge and should be mixed in a 1 : 1 ratio with water for injections before administration.
- If haloperidol is used, especially if given parenterally, anticholinergics (e.g. 1.25 mg orally (<14 years) to 2.5 mg orally (>14 years), or 2–5 mg intramuscular/intravenous (<10 years) or 5–10 mg intramuscular/ intravenous (>10 years) may also be given to reduce the risk of dystonia and other extrapyramidal side-effects. If dystonic reactions occur, anticholinergics should be administered.
- NEVER mix drugs in the same syringe.
- The advice of a consultant child and adolescent psychiatrist should be sought.
- Flumazenil (10 mcg/kg and repeat at 1 min intervals; maximum 40 mcg/kg (2 mg)) should be given if respiratory rate drops below 10

breaths per minute due to benzodiazepine administration. Repeated doses may be required as it is short acting (see current *BNF*) (although unlicensed for use in children).

- Take care when injecting a struggling child/adolescent as an intravenous bolus can result.
- Polypharmacy within a class of medicines should be avoided.
- Flumazenil is best avoided in patients with epilespsy – start mechanical ventilation instead.
- Now that there is more clinical experience using intramuscular olanzepine, this is now regarded as a more appropriate choice of intramuscular antipsychotic medication, particularly in children/ adolescents with a history of severe dystonic reactions and in those whose history is unknown or are antipsychotic naïve.
- Nursing observations should include constant visual observations, blood pressure, pulse, temperature, respiratory rate, oxygen pressure and consciousness.

Children/adolescents who are physically unwell

Avoid benzodiazepines (use antipsychotics instead) in children/adolescents who have significant respiratory impairment. Use benzodiazepines in preference to antipsychotics in patients with cardiac disease, as these are safer, but beware of accumulation.

Feedback

- The reason for prescribing any medication for the acutely disturbed child/adolescent should be documented in the medical notes, as well as the working diagnosis.
- Any medication administered to the child/adolescent and the response should be recorded in the medical notes.
- Nursing and medical staff should have a feedback session following emergency restraint and sedation.
- After the treatment of an acute disturbance, the child/adolescent should be given the opportunity to talk to a member of staff and be given an explanation of events. This should be documented in their notes and they should be offered the opportunity to write an account in their notes.
- After the treatment of an acute disturbance, the staff should also discuss the management and treatment given to the child/adolescent with the parents/carers. This discussion should be documented in the child's/adolescents' medical notes.

Further reading

American Academy of Pediatrics (1997) The use of physical restraint interventions for children and adolescents in the acute care setting. *Pediatrics*, **99**, 497–498.

Lambrenos, K. & McArthur, E. (2003) Introducing a clinical holding policy. *Paediatric Nursing*, **15**, 30–33.

Royal College of Nursing (2003) *Restraining, Holding Still and Containing Young Children and Young People*. Royal College of Nursing (http://www.rcn.org.uk/__data/assets/ pdf_file/0009/78570/001999.pdf).

Royal Liverpool Children's NHS Trust (2005) *Clinical Holding Policy*. Royal Liverpool Children's NHS Trust (http://www.alderhey.org.uk/data/documents/ ClinicalHoldingPolicy.pdf).

CHAPTER 7

Consent, capacity and mental health legislation

Mary Mitchell

The following chapter has been written with particular reference to England and Wales. The legal frameworks in Scotland and in Ireland are different, but in general the principles applied are similar.

Consent to treatment and hospital admission

Definition

Consent is the voluntary and continuing permission of a patient to receive a particular treatment, based on adequate knowledge of the purpose, nature, likely effects and risks of that treatment, including the likelihood of its success and any alternatives to it.

For consent to be valid, the young person must have:

- information about the treatment proposed:
    - that would be recognised as sufficient by a responsible body of colleagues (the Bolam Test);
    - that addresses the purpose, nature, likely effects and risks of that treatment, including the likelihood of its success and any alternatives to it;
    - that is pitched at the right level, i.e. explained in a way most likely to be understood by the patient, taking into account the young person's language, culture and age.
- the capacity (for those of 16 or over) or competence (for young people under 16) to make the decision (see below);
- free choice (not to feel coerced by others or by the circumstances).

Terminology

- Capacity is a legal term (derived from the Mental Capacity Act 2005) which applies only to people aged 16 or over.
- Competence (Gillick competence) is the equivalent legal term (derived from the Children Act 1989) for the younger person (under 16).

- In Scotland, the Age of Legal Capacity (Scotland) Act 1991 would apply.

Capacity to make treatment decisions: young people ≥ 16 years

It has been accepted for a considerable time that the consent of anyone 16 years or older to any surgical, medical or dental treatment is as effective as it would be if they were 'of full age' and it has not been necessary to obtain consent for the treatment from their parent or guardian (Family Law Reform Act 1969 Section 8.) The Mental Capacity Act 2005, which became operational in October 2007, clarifies some of the grey areas of consent to treatment and establishes clearly the principle that everyone aged 16 or over shall be presumed to have the capacity to make decisions, unless shown not to have capacity. It provides a definition of incapacity (Section 2) that:

> 'a person (16+) lacks capacity in relation to a matter if at the material time he is unable to make a decision for himself in relation to the matter because of an impairment of, or a disturbance in the functioning of, the mind or brain.'

To establish incapacity, the following two steps should be addressed.

- Is there an impairment of or a disturbance in the functioning of the person's mind or brain?
- Is that impairment or disturbance sufficient to make the person unable to make the decision in question?

Testing capacity

Can the young person, at the time the treatment is proposed:

- understand the information relevant to the question;
- retain the information for long enough to make the decision;
- use or weigh that information as part of the process of making the decision;
- communicate their decision?

Application

The most common situation in emergency departments is perhaps the patient who refuses treatment following an overdose. The principle of a presumption of capacity is established in the Mental Capacity Act 2005, therefore the decision of a patient (who is 16 or over) to refuse treatment should be presumed to be a decision made with capacity unless the clinician suspects that the patient lacks the capacity to make such a decision. It will be the clinician's responsibility to demonstrate incapacity according to the tests outlined above and to document their reasoning in the medical file.

When making an assessment of incapacity in such situations, it is worth remembering that a disturbance of or an impairment in the functioning of the mind or brain could be caused by drugs, alcohol, agitation and mental disorder in its broadest sense. Also, the IQ of the patient or any concomitant developmental difficulties may impair their ability to understand information provided. Difficulties with attention and concentration that occur in many psychiatric disorders or highly charged emotional states may have an effect on the young person's ability to retain information. Emotional immaturity, thinking that has become delusional, obsessional or nihilistic, and a disregard for future consequences will have a significant ability on a young person's ability to weigh information. Finally, a patient who is comatose, psychomotor retarded, catatonic or with severe social communication difficulties may not be able to communicate their decision. Problems in any of these areas may leave a patient incapable of making the decision at the time, once the clinician has taken all practicable steps to enable the patient to make the decision.

The Code of Practice (Section 12.13) to the Mental Capacity Act 2005 (Department for Constitutional Affairs, 2007) also includes a statement that:

> 'even where a young person (16 or 17) is presumed to have legal capacity to consent to treatment, they may not necessarily be able to make the relevant decision ... for example because they are overwhelmed by the implications of the decision, the Act will not apply to them and the legality of any treatment should be assessed under common law principles.'

Therefore, for example, in the case of the young person aged 16 or 17 refusing treatment for overdose, the clinician will need to carefully assess if the young person has the capacity to refuse, and if so, then to consider whether or not they are 'overwhelmed by the implications of the decision'. In the latter case, proceeding with treatment under common law remains an option within the law.

Competence to make treatment decisions: young people <16 years

A younger person (under 16) may make treatment decisions without parental involvement if the admitting doctor assesses them as being competent to do so (the so-called Gillick competence), that is:

> 'if the doctor concludes that he or she has the capacity to make the decision to have the proposed treatment and is of sufficient understanding and intelligence to be capable of making up his/her own mind' (Department of Health, 2008).

The test for competence of a young person under 16 to give consent without informing the parent(s) (Fraser guidelines) includes that:

- they must understand the professional's advice;
- they cannot be persuaded to inform parents;
- they are likely to suffer with regard to their mental or physical health unless they receive the requested or proposed treatment;
- their best interests require them to receive the treatment with or without parental consent.

Assessing competence

There has been a growing tendency to use Fraser guidelines when considering the competence of a young person rather than the broader definition of Gillick competence outlined earlier, perhaps because more specific guidance has been needed.

The tests of capacity under the Mental Capacity Act 2005 (as it applies to people over the age of 16) can be used when assessing the competence of younger people. Thus, the young person, at the time of the proposed treatment, must be able to:

- understand the information relevant to the question;
- retain the information for long enough to make the decision;
- use or weigh that information as part of the process of making the decision;
- communicate their decision.

The power of parents to decide on behalf of young people

A parent with parental responsibility may make a decision about treatment and hospital admission on behalf of a child for whom they have responsibility. Under the Children Act 1989, a child is a minor up to 18 years of age, and accordingly a parent with parental responsibility will continue to hold responsibility for a young person until they are 18 years of age.

Who has parental responsibility for a young person?

- Mothers always have parental responsibility (unless displaced by a freeing order in adoption proceedings).
- The child's father and mother both have parental responsibility if married at the time of the child's birth.
- Parental responsibility may in some circumstances also fall to the (unmarried) father, step-parents, other 'statutory' parents or the Local Authority (Box 7.1).

What if urgent intervention is needed?

If the parents are not available or there is uncertainty about their whereabouts and decisions cannot wait until they are found, then those who have care of the child or adolescent may intervene.

> 'A person who does not have parental responsibility for a particular child but has care of the child may do what is reasonable in all the circumstances of the case for the purpose of safeguarding or promoting the child's welfare.' (Children Act 1989 Section 3.5)

Parents' right to overrule treatment refusal by a young person

According to Mr Justice Thorpe's ruling (*Re W* [1992]), 'a child with Gillick competence can consent to treatment, but if he or she declines to

---

Box 7.1 How can parental responsibility be acquired?

Father (not married to the mother of the child)
- Named on birth certificate after December 2004
- Registration
- Formal agreement with the mother
- Court order

Step-parents
- Formal agreement with the mother
- Court order

Other 'statutory' parents
- Special guardianship
- Residence order (the holder of a residence order shares parental responsibility)
- Adoption

Local Authority shares parental responsibility if the child is under:
- an interim or full care order
- a secure order
- an emergency protection order

---

do so, consent can be given by someone (else) who has parental rights and responsibilities'.

The law in England and Wales at the moment, but not in Scotland, considers the refusal of treatment by a minor to be a more difficult decision than consent to treatment. In Scotland, if the young person is deemed competent, they can withhold as well as give consent to treatment. There is a trend towards this position in the rest of the UK now, with new mental health and capacity legislation and practice guidance in England and Wales discouraging the treatment of competent young people against their wishes. Furthermore, the scope of decisions a parent can make in overruling a competent child are now more clearly demarcated. Thus, a parent can give consent only to treatment/intervention considered to be 'within the zone of parental control' (something a parent would normally have authority over as judged by the standards of their community) and as long as there are no grounds for suspecting that the parent will not act in the child's interest (Code of Practice Mental Health Act 1983; Department of Health, 2008: pp. 329–331). (This limitation applies also to parental consent for a young person of 16 or 17 who lacks capacity.)

The Mental Capacity Act 2005 now provides clear guidance on the circumstances when decisions may be made in the best interests of patients aged 16 and over who lack capacity and are refusing treatment, and the limits to such power. If treatment amounting to a deprivation of liberty is the necessary intervention for a young patient of any age with mental disorder then it would be appropriate to consider a Mental Health Act 1983 Assessment. In effect, a parent can oblige a child to be in a hospital, but if the child actively tries to leave, cannot be persuaded to stay and needs (or would need) to be restrained to make them stay, this amounts to deprivation of liberty and the Mental Health Act should be applied if staying is imperative to protect their or other's safety. There is no lower age limit for the use of the Mental Health Act in these circumstances. The safeguards for a patient 16–18 are already defined in the Children Act 1989 in the secure accommodation order Section 25 (see *Secure accommodation order (Children Act 1989 Section 25)*, pp. 96–97).

Legal principles and frameworks in the emergency treatment of young people

The laws that are relevant in the UK are listed in Box 7.2.

Common law

English and Welsh law is based on a common law system with the application of precedents from previously tried cases, amended by statute law and European law. Treatment can be given under common law:

- according to the doctrine of necessity;
- in the best interests of the patient;
- to preserve life, health or well-being;
- to manage a crisis proportionately.

Mental Health Act 1983 and the 2007 ammendments

An assessment under the Mental Health Act 1983 (amended in 2007; see Appendix III for a brief description of the relevant Mental Health Act sections) might be the most appropriate legal framework when providing treatment and admission to hospital of young people with mental disorders.

- There is no minimum age limit for admission to hospital under the Act.

Box 7.2 Relevant laws in the UK

- Common law
- Children Act 1989 (England and Wales); 1995 (Scotland)
- Mental Health Act 1983
- The 2007 ammendments of the Mental Health Act 1983
- Mental Health (Care and Treatment) (Scotland) Act 2003
- Human Rights Act 1998
- Mental Capacity Act 2005
- Age of Legal Capacity (Scotland) Act 1991
- Social Work (Scotland) Act 1968
- Case law (judical precedent)

- The 'nearest relative' under the Mental Health Act 1983 is the older of the two parents if they both had parental responsibility. (The nearest relative may be displaced by an order of the county court by application from the approved mental health practitioner (formerly the approved social worker) or the young person or the relative themselves, if another relative would be more appropriate to hold this role.)

Although it is sometimes appropriate to use the Mental Health Act for the treatment of psychiatric illness in young people, the Code of Practice advises that consideration is given to the Children Act 1989. Guiding principles when considering use of the Mental Health Act with young people include:

- children should be kept fully informed, and their views and wishes should be taken into account;
- any intervention should be the least restrictive alternative with the least possible segregation from family, friends, community and schools;
- all children in hospital should receive appropriate education.

The Mental Health (Care and Treatment) (Scotland) Act 2003 specifically refers to human rights legislation and also spells out a series of basic principles.

All practitioners working with children are encouraged to read the relevant legislation and guidance notes for the Mental Health Act operative in their jurisdiction.

Human Rights Act 1998

It is unlawful for a public authority to act in a way which is incompatible with the European Convention on Human Rights. When making difficult decisions with parents about the care of young people there may be competing convention rights, particularly the child's right to liberty (Article 5) and the parents' right to respect for private and family life (Article 8). When deliberating the best way forward, it is important to consider which intervention best protects the interests and the human rights of the child. The clinician has a duty of care and requirement to act lawfully. The child might benefit from the statutory protection within the Mental Health Act but which is not explicit under parental responsibility. People to whom the Mental Health Act 1983 applies should none the less receive recognition of their basic human rights.

Lawful decision-making when providing treatment to young people in crisis

- Determine the 'capacity' (>16 years) or 'competence' (<16 years) of the young person to make their own decisions.

- Establish who has parental responsibility (a parent may need to know and might help in treatment decisions).
- Although it may be clinically appropriate to contact both parents, a doctor may proceed with the consent of one parent with parental responsibility only, even if the other parent objects.
- Where a parent with parental responsibility refuses consent, evaluate the reasons for this objection and the grounds on which it was made (is the parent in your view clearly acting against the child's interest?). If there is time, it may be appropriate to make an application to the court (Inherent Jurisdiction).
- Establish if the young person is mentally ill, and if so, does the severity of the disorder justify the remedy proposed (is it proportionate?).
- Consider whether the needs of the child could be better met in a Social Services or education placement (taking into account the discrimination and stigma that the young person is likely to experience if they are compulsorily detained in a mental health institution).

Hospital admission under the Mental Health Act is not appropriate for behavioural disturbance not caused by a mental disorder.

Psychiatric disorder: lawful decision-making to treat or admit[1]

Is the young person consenting to treatment and/or in-patient admission?

If yes (consenting)

- Treat and/or admit.
- Seek the young person's agreement to inform parents.
- Seek to involve parents of young people aged <16.

If no (not consenting) and under 16

- If the young person is competent and refusing, the Mental Health Act Code of Practice suggests it is unwise to treat with parental consent:
  - consider an assessment under the Mental Health Act 1983; or
  - an application to the court.
- If the young person lacks competence to make the decision, the consent of one parent (with parental responsibility) is sufficient to proceed as long as the intervention falls in the zone of parental control:
  - otherwise consider a Mental Health Act assessment or an application to the courts;
  - consider assessment under the Mental Health Act if intervention amounts to a deprivation of liberty;

---

1. See also *Code of Practice Mental Health Act 1983*, decision-making trees, pp. 350–352 (Department of Health, 2008).

- if the young person and both parents do not consent, and failure to treat/admit poses urgent and significant risks, consider using powers of the the Mental Health Act to detain for assessment (see below);
- if criteria for the Mental Health Act are not met, consider application to the court.

If no (not consenting) and 16–18

- Since the Section 131 amendment to the Mental Health Act 1983, a parent with parental responsibility cannot overrule the refusal of a young person aged 16 or over if that young person has the capacity to make the decision in question and the intervention is treatment in hospital for a mental disorder: assessment under the Mental Health Act is indicated.

Severe psychiatric disorder

Even if it is legally possible to treat a young person with parental consent, there are conditions when it might be preferable to use the Mental Health Act (see Appendix III), for example:

- inconsistent parental consent;
- doubts about the parent's motives in detaining the young person;
- statutory safeguards for the protection of the rights of the young person (i.e. right of appeal);
- where treatment amounts to a deprivation of liberty or is beyond 'the zone of parental control', for example if restraint, intramuscular injections or nasogastric feeding are required (Department of Health 2008).

Treatment of physical illness under the Mental Health Act

This is possible under the Mental Health Act, but only:

- if the physical problem is a manifestation of the mental disorder; and
- if the treatment of the physical problem is ancillary to the core treatment of the mental disorder.

For example:

- nasogastric feeding for anorexia nervosa
- overdose secondary to severe depressive illness.

A person detained under the Mental Health Act may still have capacity to refuse medical treatment that is not treatment covered by the Act itself. This capacity has to be assessed in relation to the treatment proposed. Capacity is not a global attribution, but specific to the decision to be made.

Treating the medical consequences of self-harm

This issue according to the law is not the severity of the 'injury', but the capacity of the patient to make treatment decisions and the circumstances that allow a patient's decision to be overruled with impunity.

The authority to treat the consequences of self-harm may come from the following.

- The consent of the patient.
- The consent of a parent with parental responsibility (or the Local Authority under a care order or the Inherent Jurisdiction of the High Court) of a young person up to the age of 16.
- After 16, if the young person is assessed as having the capacity (see Section 2 of the Mental Capacity Act 2005; see *Testing capacity*, p. 87) to make the treatment decision, their refusal of treatment should be respected even if it seems irrational.
- For 16- and 17-year-olds, if the young person is assessed as not having the capacity to make the treatment decision, treatment may proceed in the best interest of the patient, as defined in the Mental Capacity Act 2005 Code of Practice (Department for Constitutional Affairs, 2007).
- For 16- and 17-year-olds, if the young person is assessed as having capacity but is or is likely to be 'overwhelmed' by the implications of the decision, treatment may proceed under common law principles.
- If the patient is mentally ill and all the criteria for detention under the Mental Health Act are met and the treatment of the physical injury is 'ancillary to the treatment of the mental disorder', treatment may proceed under Section 63 of the Mental Health Act.[2]
- A patient cannot be detained under the Mental Health Act solely for the treatment of the physical problem. Only if the patient needs to be detained for treatment of their mental disorder and the treatment of the physical problem is treatment ancillary to the core treatment of the mental disorder can the authority of a section under the Act be used to enforce physical treatment.
- A patient who is compulsorily detained for the treatment of mental illness may still have the capacity to refuse treatment for physical illness.

---

2. The 2007 amendments to the Mental Health Act 1983 include a much broader definition of mental disorder, that is, 'any disorder or disability of the mind', and 'appropriate medical treatment' means what is appropriate in the patient's case 'for the purpose of alleviating, or preventing a worsening of the disorder or one or more of its symptoms or manifestations'. Symptoms or manifestations include the way a disorder is experienced by the individual and the way in which the disorder manifests itself in the person's thoughts, emotions, behaviour and actions. Thus, it is lawful to treat the effects of self-harm (the poisoning or the injuries) under the amended Act.

- The assessment of capacity depends on the context and the treatment decision at the time.
- When there is doubt about a patient's capacity or competence, treatment may be provided under the common law doctrine of necessity, as long as it is:
  - in the best interests of the young person
  - to preserve life, health or well-being
  - proportionate to the degree of harm.

Behavioural disturbance without formal psychiatric disorder

If, following assessment, there is no evidence of mental disorder and psychiatric treatment under compulsion is not necessary, the following should be considered.

- What are the risk factors?
- How can the risk be reduced?
- Short-term plans need regular review.
- Secure accommodation order (under the Children Act 1989 Section 25).

Secure accommodation order (Children Act 1989 Section 25)

In order to apply for a secure accommodation order, the young person should:

- have a history of absconding;
- is likely to abscond from any other description of accommodation;
- if they abscond, they are likely to suffer significant harm.

    OR

- If kept in any other description of accommodation, the young person is likely to injure themselves or others.
- A child who meets the criteria may be placed in secure accommodation for a maximum period of 72 h in any 28-day period without court authority.
- Applications to the director of Social Services.
- If under 13 years, apply to the Home Secretary (in England).

A secure accommodation order is not usually available in an acute crisis. This option could be discussed with the duty social worker, who may be reticent about applying to the court for a secure order in an emergency situation, especially out of hours, without a detailed and comprehensive social assessment. However, this is worth considering as part of a crisis plan for the small number of adolescents who attend the emergency department frequently, especially from social care placements, where previous assessments have pointed to a conduct disorder, rather than formal mental illness, as the main organising problem underlying their repeated attendance in the emergency department, often with minor or threatened self-harm, and especially when previous admissions to a mental health unit had made the problem worse rather than better, which is sometimes the case.

Substance misuse and dependency

Substance misuse and dependency is not deemed to be a disorder of the mind for the purposes of the Mental Health Act. Thus, it is not lawful to detain someone under the Mental Health Act because they are dependent on substances (drugs or alcohol) or to manage detoxification, unless they are also suffering from a mental disorder (e.g. psychosis or severe depression), the safe treatment of which requires hospitalisation.

Acute intoxication and/or its complications are best treated (without the patient's consent) under common law or as allowed under the Mental Capacity Act.

Intellectual disability

It is possible to detain someone with intellectual disability in hospital under a treatment order of the Mental Health Act, only:

• if they have a mental disorder that meets the criteria for detention;
• if they are dangerously aggressive or seriously irresponsible.

It is not lawful to detain a person with intellectual disability for the purposes of treating the intellectual disability itself, in the absence of the above qualifications.

CHAPTER 8

Child abuse and child protection

Tricia Brennan

Safeguarding and promoting the welfare of children is the responsibility of all health staff. It involves protecting children from harm, preventing impairment of children's health or development, and ensuring all children are growing up in circumstances consistent with the provision of safe and effective care.

Child protection is part of safeguarding children and involves all forms of maltreatment of a child. Somebody may abuse or neglect a child by inflicting harm or by failing to prevent harm. Children may be abused in a family, or in institutional or community settings, by those known to them, or more rarely, by a stranger. It is important to realise that parental problems such as mental ill health, intellectual difficulties, substance (including alcohol) misuse and domestic violence can impact on an adult's parenting ability and therefore affect their child.

The UK government defines a child in this context as anyone below the age of 18 years.

Types of abuse

Four main categories of abuse have been defined; physical abuse, neglect, emotional abuse and sexual abuse, although in some cases it is difficult to categorise the abuse. It is important to note that if a child suffers one type, then they are likely to have also suffered other types and thus the assessment must include all aspects of the child.

Physical abuse includes assaults such as hitting, shaking, poisoning and burning or scalding. It also includes fabricated and induced illness.

Neglect is the persistent failure to meet a child's basic physical and/ or psychological needs, likely to result in the serious impairment of the child's health or development. It includes failure to take the child for appropriate medical care. It can begin in pregnancy when the mother misuses substances.

Emotional abuse is the persistent emotional maltreatment of a child such as to cause severe and persistent adverse effects of the child's emotional development, making the child feel unloved and inadequate. It can include bullying or corrupting a child, or seeing or hearing the ill treatment of another person such as in domestic violence.

Sexual abuse involves forcing or enticing a child or adolescent to take part in sexual activities, whether or not they are aware of the implications.

The (long-term) effects of child abuse can be many and varied. Each type of abuse can have effects on the child's physical development. Abuse can have an effect on attachment and lead to difficulties in developing and sustaining relationships, behavioural difficulties including withdrawal or aggression, risk-taking behaviour, poor self-esteem, depression, PTSD, and difficulties in regulating affect, with angry and/or self-destructive behaviour and substance misuse. The child or adolescent may, therefore, present to an emergency department with behavioural, psychological and/or psychiatric problems.

The government produced *Working Together to Safeguard Children* in 2006 (HM Governement, 2006). This publication sets out the responsibilities and duties of staff from many agencies, including health, in safeguarding children and child protection. All health staff are expected to know the indicators of abuse, and know how to manage suspected cases within their own organisation, how to refer for a multi-agency assessment, fulfilling their own role within this.

The Royal College of Paediatrics and Child Health (2006) published the *Child Protection Companion* – guidelines for recognition, investigation and management of child abuse. This is more detailed and extensive than this chapter, and should be regarded as the standard to be achieved in the training of doctors regularly working with children and adolescents.

Presentations

Child abuse or neglect may present to hospital in a number of different ways.

- Overt presentation for assessment or treatment of established abuse (non-accidental physical injury, neglect, emotional or sexual abuse).
- Abuse or neglect may be suspected as an underlying (covert) cause of the medical or emotional–behavioural problem.
- Concerns may develop while an unrelated condition is being managed.
- A child may be at risk from the behaviour or condition of an adult in the household; it may be the adult who is the patient.
- There may be concern about risk to the unborn child.
- Staff may witness abuse or neglect towards a patient or visitor.
- There may be disclosure from the child, the abuser or another party.
- Self-harm is a common presenting problem in adolescents who are being, or have been, abused.

Physical abuse

History

- Incompatible with injury
- Inconsistent, changing history
- Absent history
- Delay in presentation
- Previous concerning or frequent attendances

Examination

- Injuries of different ages
- Incompatible with child's age/development/ability
- Unusual site (e.g. soft, protected areas of body such as neck or inner arms)
- Unusual shape or pattern (e.g. parallel linear bruises)
- Injuries suggesting self-harm (e.g. linear scars to elbows/wrists)

Neglect

- Failure of care leading to significant impairment of the child's health, development or well-being
- Failure to protect the child form exposure to danger
- Failure to provide or maintain recommended medical treatment, leading to a predictable deterioration in the child's health

Emotional abuse

- Rejection/hostility of child by family member(s)
- Gross inconsistency in parent's management of the child
- Developmentally inappropriate expectations
- Exposure to violence (the mother may be the presenting patient)
- Involvement in interparental conflict

Sexual abuse

- Pregnancy in a minor
- Perineal/urinary symptoms and/or signs
- Sexually transmitted disease
- Recurrent abdominal pain/headaches
- Child hinting at undisclosed secrets
- Mental health presentations such as depression or self-harm
- Inappropriate sexual knowledge
- Sexualised behaviour
- Eccentric sexualised patterns of family interaction
- Self-harm

Vulnerable groups

Special consideration needs to be given to the risk in the following groups.

- Younger children
- Socially excluded families
- Domestic violence between the adult carers
- Mental health problems in parents/carers
- Parents/carers misusing drugs/alcohol
- Chronically ill or disabled children
- Child prostitutes
- A history of abuse in the parent's childhood (although it is the minority (about 30%) of abuse survivors who will become abusive towards children in their care)
- History of abuse to another child of either parent

Parental problems and child protection

Mental ill health or substance misuse in a parent or carer does not necessarily have a negative impact on a child, but it is essential to assess the implications for all children in the immediate family. Parental illness may restrict the child's social and recreational activities. Parents with depression may neglect the child's physical and emotional needs. A significant burden of care within the household may fall upon the child and this should be assessed.

If the parent or carer is misusing drugs or alcohol, the best care in many cases for the child will be in the context of full support for the parent.

Management: child protection procedure

If a professional is concerned that a child is at risk of or has suffered significant harm through abuse, they need to be guided by their local child protection procedures. Junior staff should always discuss the case with their seniors. The trust in which the doctor works may have a child protection team, including named doctors for child protection/safeguarding, who may also be a source of advice. If it is agreed that there is concern, a referral should be made to Social Services.

Sexual activity involving a child under 13 years of age should always be discussed with the nominated child protection lead of the organisation and a referral to Social Services should be made. Sexual activity in 13- to 15-year-olds may also be of concern, and should not be automatically dismissed as 'normal' for that age. In the case of a young person aged 13–15 years, where the sexual relationship is consensual between non-related young people and the age differential is not substantial, the decision to refer to Social Services may be more difficult. Significant harm should be the guiding principle, for example with regard to risk taking, exploitation, effects on self-esteem, prostitution, etc. Cases should be discussed with the consultant and with the child protection lead if necessary.

If a professional is concerned that a child may be at risk of or have suffered significant harm, they should:

- acknowledge their concerns
- discuss their concerns with a senior/more experienced professional
- ensure the child is safe
- refer to other services such as social care services, according to local guidelines
- play a proper role in further assessment (e.g. prepare reports/ attend case conferences on request)
- help to define further treatment as appropriate.

Ensuring the child's safety and well-being

The hospital as a place of safety

There are occasions when a child is admitted to hospital when there is no medical or nursing need, because of a risk of harm. The hospital acts as a place of safety for the child. Social Services should give careful consideration to other placements such as foster care or other family members.

When in the hospital, a robust plan should be in place including:

- visiting/contact restrictions
- supervision of contact between child and others, including family members
- legal orders in place if necessary
- police involvement
- contact numbers for involved professionals such as the consultant paediatrician, social worker or child abuse police unit
- regular review dates
- discharge planning.

Using the law to protect children

Public law

There are several measures that can be taken in order to protect children.

Police protection

A police constable can remove a child to a safe place or prevent the removal of a child from a safe place if the officer believes that the child is suffering or likely to suffer significant harm if action is not taken. It is usually taken in an emergency situation. It does not confer parental responsibility on police or Social Services.

Emergency protection order

The Local Authority can apply to a court for this order, usually in an urgent situation, if it believes a child would suffer from or be likely to suffer from significant harm if the child was not removed from where they are or kept in a particular place (e.g. in a hospital). Whoever is granted the order, usually the Local Authority, acquires parental responsibility for the duration of the order (i.e. 8 days which can be extended by a further 7 days).

Care orders

Only the Local Authority and the charity National Society for the Prevention of Cruelty to Children can apply for a care order if:

- the child is suffering from or at risk of suffering from significant harm;
- the harm is likely to be due to the care being given to them or is beyond parental control.

The order does confer parental responsibility on the Local Authority, which shares it with the parents.

Supervision order

A supervision order can be made if a court decides there is sufficient concern for a child to be supervised. It does not confer parental responsibility on the Local Authority.

Both care orders and supervision orders can be made on an interim basis while there are ongoing preparations for the court's final hearing.

Private law

The court can make various orders in private law which may be used according to the individual needs of the child.

Residence order

It confers parental responsibility to the person with the benefit of the residence order and it states with whom the child is to live.

Contact order

This requires the person with whom the child lives to allow the child to have contact with the persons named in the order.

Prohibited steps order

This prevents the parents of a child taking any steps in meeting their authority of the kind stated in the order without first obtaining the permission of the court.

Consent

Consent must be given for assessment and examination of a child, although implied consent is usually assumed for out-patient-type consultation.

In children where there are child protection concerns, it is preferable to use a consent form, which is an integral part of the pro forma used for examining the child. Consent for examination for anyone under 16 should be sought from someone with parental responsibility.

It is important for doctors and other health professionals to establish who can give parental consent before assessing and treating a child (see Chapter 7). Foster carers have *de facto* parental responsibility if a child in their care is under a care order (although technically the director of Social Services holds this authority under the law, and devolves the execution of this to the allocated social worker), but neither the foster carer nor the Local Authority has it if the child has been placed in foster care as a voluntary arrangement ('accommodated'). Parental responsibility diminishes with increasing age and independence of a child.

A young person under 16 years of age may be judged to be Gillick competent and is able to take some decisions for themselves. A young person over 16 is deemed competent (capacitous) unless demonstrably otherwise.

Training and support

- All professional staff working with children and adolescents under 18 should have training in safeguarding children to enable them to fulfil their professional responsibilities.
- All staff working with children and adolescents under 18 should be aware of, and have access to, written copies of their locally agreed child protection procedures.
- All staff working with children and adolescents under 18 should know who the designated lead for child protection is for their discipline within their organisation.
- This work can be difficult and staff need to know where to go for professional and sometimes personal advice and support – this may initially be a senior in their own organisation, or a designated or nominated professional.

Role of emergency department staff in child protection

As the first point of contact, the emergency department has a crucial role in the detection and management of the abused child.

In the history taking, the following points must be noted:

- the timescale between injury and attendance
- the compatibility and consistency between injury and history given
- the parent–child, parent–staff and child–staff interactions
- relevant previous attendances and those of siblings
- child protection register list check.

In the examination, the careful and accurate documentation of all injuries is of particular importance. Any disclosure of abuse should be recorded verbatim; you should ask open questions and record both the question and the answer. The parents'/carers' statements, responses and their behaviour towards and relationship with their child (and the child's responses) should be documented. It is important that the immensely challenging context of being suspected of child abuse should be taken into account in evaluating these observations.

The help of the most senior paediatrician must be sought immediately – examination should be carefully detailed, performed and carried out by an experienced clinician. The assessment should be holistic; issues of emotional and sexual abuse and neglect, as well as of physical abuse, should be considered.

If there are concerns, the input of a senior clinician should be sought, and if the concern remains, the child should be admitted under the care of the paediatrician.

If a concern remains but is below the threshold of concern requiring immediate protection, a 'cause for concern' system should alert the relevant practitioner (e.g. school nurse, health visitor) about the current presentation.

Emergency department staff must have guidelines, training and support with regard to child protection to enable them to:

- identify where there are child protection concerns in children;
- undertake an assessment of the child to gather more information for other professionals;
- be able to deal sensitively (but if necessary firmly) with parents suspected of abuse;
- discuss the concerns with a senior professional;
- refer to the paediatric on-take team for further child assessment.

Role of paediatric staff in child protection

The paediatric team should do a further assessment of the case. This will include:

- a full top-to-toe examination looking for injuries but also for general signs such as cleanliness, growth, demeanour and a brief developmental check;
- any investigations, for example skeletal survey and computerised tomography scan in young infants who have other injuries;
- checks with the health visitor or GP to identify whether there are any known concerns about the child or the family and to check the child is not the subject of a child protection plan;
- referral to Social Services if there are any child protection concerns;
- work with social workers to ensure the child is in a safe place while

the multi-agency child protection investigation (Children Act 1989 Section 47) takes place.

Role of CAMHS in child protection[1]

In the course of their work, child and adolescent mental health professionals will want to identify as part of their assessment and care planning whether child abuse, neglect or domestic violence are factors in a child's mental health problems and to ensure they are addressed appropriately in the treatment and care delivered. If the mental health professional thinks a child is currently affected, they should follow the child protection procedures laid down for their services within their area. Consultation, supervision and training resources for child protection procedures should be available and accessible in each service.

Child and adolescent mental health professionals have a role in the initial assessment process in children in whom child abuse is suspected in circumstances where their specific skills and knowledge are helpful. Examples include:

- children and adolescents with severe behavioural and emotional disturbance;
- eating disorder or self-harming behaviour;
- families where there is a perceived high risk of danger;
- very young children;
- where the abused child or abuser has severe communication problems;
- where the parent or carer fabricate or induce illness;
- where multiple victims are involved.

In addition, assessment and treatment services may need to be provided to young people with mental health problems who conduct criminal offences.

The assessment of children with significant learning difficulties, a disability, or sensory and communication difficulties, may require the expertise of a CAMHS or specialist learning disability service.

Child and adolescent mental health services also have a role in the provision of a range of psychiatric and psychological assessment and treatment services for children and families. Services that may be provided in liaison with Social Services include the provision of reports for court, and direct work with children, parents and families. Services may be provided either within general or specialist multidisciplinary teams, depending upon the severity and complexity of the problem. In addition, consultation and training may be offered to services in the community including, for example, Social Services, schools, primary healthcare teams and nurseries.

---

1. Taken from *Working Together to Safeguard Children* (HM Governement, 2006; pp. 58–59).

CHAPTER 9

Cultural diversity and mental health problems

Begum Maitra

Epidemiological studies suggest that certain psychiatric disorders are diagnosed more frequently in some ethnic groups (Malek & Joughin, 2004). However, the multifactorial aetiologies of these conditions, and the problems inherent in how ethnicity is defined, suggest caution in how we interpret the links between them. Although the lack of a biological basis to 'race' has led to the contemporary focus on 'ethnicity' as a way of identifying cultural differences, ethnic categories are based on such dissimilar criteria[1] that they tell us little about which factors may be relevant to the emotionally/behaviourally disturbed child or adolescent.

However, some vulnerability factors are particularly relevant to children and families from ethnic minority groups. These include stressors arising from the contexts and process of migration (complex bereavement and dislocation), from experiences of discrimination, and as a result of differential rates of acculturation between the first and second generation. Other factors contribute to delay in presentation at health services – different expectations of services, communication difficulties, suspicion of statutory services and a belief that services will not be sensitive or respectful to the family's cultural beliefs.

Whatever the case may be, as with young people from ethnic/cultural majority groups, presentation at a hospital emergency department usually follows a crisis in the life of the child/family, and skilled assessment is necessary to establish the health priorities at this point – cultural factors may or may not be relevant to the decisions that need to be made. Despite this, a culturally competent assessment remains central to an understanding of the child's context and their presentation in hospital.

---

1. As the ethnic categories used by the Office of National Statistics show, these are based on widely differing criteria that elide geography with morphology, religion and 'political' intention, for example: the terms White and Black Caribbean seem to refer to skin 'colour' and geographical region; 'Indian', 'Pakistani' and 'Bangladeshi' refer to national boundaries, and perhaps to religious difference among people with very similar cultures; unclear terms such as Asian that have no specific reference point, and mean different things elsewhere.

Assessment

It is essential under such circumstances to take an accurate history that includes an understanding of the cultural background. All the basic principles of good history taking apply, but these need to be supported by a framework that facilitates cultural enquiry and discussion.

The family context

A systematic enquiry into the context of the child's/adolescent's difficulties must ensure that a range of views are obtained. It is important to resist the temptation to accept the most easily comprehensible version; namely, that of the person whose language or point of view is most familiar. In families from ethnic minority groups this is often the view of the child/ adolescent presenting with difficulties (or a sibling). Although careful attention needs to be paid to their account, it is important to bear in mind that the 'voice of the child' must be placed in the context of other views, namely those of adults within that family/cultural group. Every attempt must be made to interview the main carer/legal parent, and to obtain their thoughts about the problem and of potential solutions. This can sometimes be difficult when children explicitly request that their parents not be informed of their difficulties, or when the parent is presented as the 'cause' of the young person's distress. Emotional and cognitive immaturity may contribute to children's/adolescent's perceptions of a parent, and to a misunderstanding of parental intention. Although this may be true for parent–child conflict in all cultures, error in gauging the nature and seriousness of such conflicts are more likely to arise when there is significant cultural difference between the patient/family and the professional making the assessment.

Clarity of communication across cultural/linguistic differences

Families arriving from countries with different constructs regarding emotions and emotional problems (and mental illness), and with different socio-legal structures to address childhood problems, may have little understanding of the premises of British health and social care systems. Their capacity to comprehend differences of this sort will be further undermined by the highly stressful circumstances of accompanying a seriously unwell/disturbed child to the emergency department, a difficulty that is exacerbated by family members' non-fluency in English, the primary language of assessment.

Using interpreters

Effective communication is vital in order to make a mental health assessment, and it is essential to address the language problems of a young patient and/ or their family members who are unable to communicate fully in English. This needs to be addressed, where possible, by having the assessment made by a competent mental health professional who is also proficient in the patient's language, an option that is unfortunately rarely feasible in an emergency situation. Next best and usually more easily available, is to engage a well-trained interpreter, if possible a 'link worker', a specially designated interpreter, well-acquainted with the family's culture who can also act as a patient/family advocate. Interpreters, to be of most use in the assessment of complex mental health and relational problems, should have had prior training in mental health issues. This avoids the problem of interpreters being reluctant to or failing to translate speech seen as 'rubbish', 'nonsense', 'rude' or worse. However, it is important to remember that concepts in one language are not always open to simple translation into another, however skilled the interpreter. It is never good practice to rely on a family member, especially a child in the family (even though the children are often more proficient in English) to interpret.

It should be recognised that the interpreter's task is complicated by factors that may discourage the family from disclosing their concerns openly. For example, there may be differences in dialect, intracultural variation due to region, class or religion that the interpreter is unfamiliar with, or conflicts within the cultural community, for example, tensions due to the family and interpreter belonging to different ideological/political factions. A preliminary discussion with the interpreter to consider how these difficulties might be broached will assist the doctor in weighing up the quality of information available at interview.

Furthermore, the interpreter and the doctor need to find a way of indicating the subtle shifts in mood, motivation and cooperation, or ambiguity in verbal/non-verbal expression that are vital information if the doctor is not to base important decisions about the nature and seriousness of the problem on inaccurate data.

What is less widely acknowledged are the particular personal and professional skills necessary in the assessing professional. They will require a great deal of patience, persistence and flexibility to ensure that information given and obtained is as clear as possible. A great deal of the treatment plan will depend on ensuring that the family understands the choices and decisions they will be required to make about their child's welfare.

Cultural competence

A large number of assumptions about what is 'culturally sensitive' practice appear to handicap rather than aid assessment. The basic misunderstanding is that 'respect' for cultural diversity requires one not to question facts presented by the family as religious or 'cultural' beliefs/ practices. Although some families may use cultural difference to deflect questions into areas they consider to be private, it is necessary to bear in mind that the culture one has grown up in oneself appears so normal and unremarkable as to be difficult to describe to another.

Children from ethnic minority groups and those with 'mixed' ethnicity (often referred to as 'dual heritage') grow up simultaneously in more than one culture. They are faced with the unenviable task of making sense of the contradictions this throws up, and of the unspoken hostilities, anxieties and stereotypes that complicate intergroup relations. Parents may be unaware of or unable to assist their children with these dilemmas, leading to adverse outcomes for the child/adolescent.

Other difficulties arise when children make choices (however ill-informed or mature these may be) that run counter to the family's cultural value systems. In order to encourage open discussion of these problem areas, the assessing professional should be prepared to be transparent about the (cultural) basis of British professional beliefs about children, their needs and welfare. It is this willingness to consider the relative nature of cultural systems that promotes respect, and may convince families of the assessor's genuine wish to understand the rationale of the family's cultural system. Errors are more likely to arise from a lack of confidence or anxiety about appearing ignorant, and a consequent failure to pursue what appears at first glance to be unfamiliar and problematic parenting.

Beliefs about mental illness

Beliefs about mental illness, and indeed about the nature and origins of emotions and behaviour, are socially derived, and the metaphors used to communicate about such matters are often culture specific. Thus, for example, talk of interventions by ghosts, spirits, devils and angels do not necessarily indicate psychosis – this needs to be properly understood within its cultural belief system before its phenomenological status is determined. An understanding of such cultural systems permits the professional to negotiate within a congruent system of metaphors and is invaluable therapeutically. Without this, misunderstanding and mistrust will often develop, obstructing an effective engagement and alliance.

Further considerations

There is no simple way of preparing for the enormous range of cultural diversity that one may be presented with in the multicultural society that forms present-day Britain. It is almost easier to begin with a clear awareness of the cultural premises that underlie British professional views about children and their needs, and to make these explicit as one interviews parents about how their beliefs may differ.

Cultural identities

It may be helpful to remember that children from ethnic minority groups growing up in the UK, whatever their wishes or self-perceptions, are unlikely to have single, or even simple, alliances with their cultures of origin or with mainstream British culture. The cultural identities of these children/

adolescents are more likely to be multiple, fluid and situation specific. Thus, the South Asian adolescent who is in conflict with her parents because she wishes to adopt British/Western modes of dress may wish to fit in with one significant collective (*viz.* the peer group at school), but have strong alliances with other collectives (the culturally homogeneous peer group at the temple/mosque). Despite this choice, she may have little intention to adopt other, related Western value systems (e.g. that link dress with behavioural expressions of gender roles, sexuality or other expressions of autonomous choice).

Cultural conflict

The notion of cultural conflict between parents and their children is rarely the simple matter it is often presented as – namely, in the form of polarisations between the child's 'individual' nature and its expression in choice (often viewed as Westernised, modern and progressive), and the parent's collective cultural traditions. The representation of 'the cultural tradition' as potentially coercive and harmful to the developing child's individuality is likely to be a product of the cultural biases of the (culturally) British observer. Guaranteed sufficient material resources, children across the world seem to do fairly well under a wide cultural variety of child-rearing, parenting contexts. Furthermore, there is a great deal of intracultural variation within groups, and how individual parents in the UK negotiate choices within multicultural communities is not apparent until specific questions have been addressed about parenting goals and strategies.

Discrimination

Accounts from individuals from ethnic minority groups about their cultures and cultural choices, and their attitudes towards British culture, are likely to be influenced by experiences of discrimination. It is important to remember that these may be triggered by inaccurate perceptions of the child's/family's 'ethnicity' (by their appearance or dress), and perceptions of their cultural practices by other groups (e.g. White British, as well as other ethnic minority and religious/cultural groups). In response to this, children from ethnic minority groups may or may not wish not to identify themselves as belonging to their cultures of origin, or as 'Black'. Alternatively, they may cluster in exclusive groups, avoiding other ethnic/White British peers, sometimes masking the distress of cumulative discriminatory experiences with a verbal/behavioural overlay of apparent aggression, unwittingly escalating the hostility they provoke among mainstream peers and adults such as teachers.

Emotional communication

Cultural differences in styles of emotional expression are among the most confounding variables when assessing the quality of family interaction and relationships. Evaluation of non-verbal behaviour is a vital part of assessment of the individual, and of interpersonal behaviour. What is considered 'appropriate' (polite, reasonable, cooperative) emotional expression in content, style and 'volume' varies with gender and social class, as well as culture. For example, a young person holding eye contact with an adult may be regarded as disrespectful in African Caribbean cultural tradition, whereas the opposite assumption would usually be made by most in the majority culture. Although some aspects are obviously open to conscious modification, spontaneous emotional expression in situations of high stress are less likely to be under the voluntary, or conscious, control of the individual. Equally, the gendered nature of social roles, responsibilities and behaviour become part of an individual's unconscious repertoire of choices.

Simple conclusions about parental commitment, or the quality of interpersonal relationships between parents or other family members, may not be accurate across cultural divides. For example, the South Asian doctor in the emergency department may inaccurately interpret the White British parent's emphasis on their child's autonomy as emotional coldness and disengagement, or the African parent's open (and apparently unrestrained) expression of anger towards their child may not indicate violent intention. In many cultures it is expected that male elders will take the lead in the public sphere. Fathers, who may have little to do with childcare, will often act as the main respondent, with the mother remaining silent out of respect for her husband's authority unless invited to speak by him. Her silence in this context should not be taken to mean she is submissive or oppressed in other contexts, for example with regard to child-care decision-making. Only closer skilled enquiry will reveal the quality of the parent–child and parent–parent relationships, and form the context of an accurate assessment of the risks and possibilities at hand.

Child protection

With child protection in mind, the question of whether certain cultural practices are unquestionably harmful to children is a complex one. Skilled assessment in the emergency department can contribute valuable information to these complex considerations of risk. It is essential to bear in mind that the child's/adolescent's needs and welfare are paramount, and that one of the immediate priorities is to ensure the continuing safety of the child/adolescent in question. Both under- and overestimation of risk have serious adverse consequences for the long-term welfare of the child and their position within their family and cultural group. Where parental wishes appear to pose a direct medical/emotional risk, cultural priorities must come second to considerations of the child's safety, notwithstanding the 'Western' cultural basis upon which these judgements must inevitably rest at this point. The distress and anxiety this is likely to cause parents must be treated seriously and with compassion, and sufficient explanation given about professional reasons for believing the proposed cultural practice to be harmful to the child.

Stigma

It is important to remember that the stigma associated with mental illness is not a feature of non-Western cultures alone, a great deal having been written about the effects of diagnostic 'labelling' and the negative impact on the life chances of the mentally ill in Western countries. The negative associations to mental illness can be understood by considering the cultural explanatory model, its beliefs about aetiology, outcomes and consequences. These may range from notions of physical/genetic inheritance to 'inheritance' of a spiritual/moral sort; from imbalance in diet to imbalance in the moral sphere; and from interpersonal trauma to trauma mediated through magical/supernatural means. Thus, parents who wish to take their behaviourally disturbed child to a spiritual healer are not intending to deprive them of (Western) treatment, but are interpreting the meaning and significance of the child's behaviour very differently from that of the doctor worrying about, say, early-onset psychosis. Expert opinion in both cultural camps is likely to be equally immovable on what is in the child's best interests.

Again, it is important for the doctor to carefully consider the medical/ psychiatric evidence, and to explain the seriousness of their concerns to the parents. Most parents in these circumstances are intensely anxious about their child, rather than merely ignorant or solely focused on cultural priorities. The doctor's skill at this point lies in clear explanation of immediate risks and the essential biomedical interventions necessary to prevent these. The reassurance that cultural practices may be performed concurrently, or may be introduced at a slightly later date (if satisfied that these practices do not include the use of substances or procedures that might pose other risks to the child), will go a long way to reassure and build trust with parents.

Religious belief

The child's/family's religious affiliations are not usually in themselves relevant to an assessment of mental health need. However, in some circumstances it may be important to establish which religion, if any, the patient observes. It should be borne in mind that some families may not practice their religious affiliation but may see it as part of their identity; others may practice selectively or belong to a religious minority group within the ethnic community. Religious beliefs are one among a number of interrelated belief systems that tell parents within the culture how to think about the welfare of their children and what the priorities are. This is not a factor restricted to ethnic minority communities alone since many Britons may not share the secular beliefs and faith in biomedicine common among doctors and child-care professionals.

The central considerations remain the same, namely that of assessing carefully the evidence for any parental belief system that might have a negative impact on the health and well-being of the child/adolescent, and of looking for ways to modify these beliefs, or alternatively looking to see ways in which the religious beliefs and organisation may provide solutions and comfort. An awareness of what is and what is not acceptable in the patient's religion is of great assistance in a holistic assessment. Some religions have specific expectations and requirements (e.g. prayer time, diet) that need to be observed. Not taking these into consideration may obstruct an effective assessment.

All religions have days of particular significance, and setting follow-up appointments on these dates may offend the religious sensibilities of the family. Although it is important to bear this in mind (multi-faith calendars with these important dates are widely available to help in planning appointments), these needs of the family must be weighed up against the urgency of the needs of the child/adolescent. Conflicting beliefs about the nature of the latter may appear to the professional to raise questions about the parents' ability to prioritise the child's needs. This is an error of cultural interpretation and, as detailed above, requires careful enquiry and repeated explanation of professional belief systems.

CHAPTER 10

Special considerations

Tony Kaplan

Emergency housing placements

If the young person you are dealing with has no home, cannot return home (the parents prohibit this), or should not return home (because of concerns about abuse or because the atmosphere and relationships in that home are deleterious to their mental health, for example where there is ongoing unresolved conflict), other housing placements will have to be considered if hospitalisation is not indicated or is not the least restrictive safe option (Box 10.1).

Returning home or to kinship housing

The assessing social worker has a duty to preserve the child's placement in their family or to look for another placement for the child, if only short term, with related kin or trusted friends known to the family whenever possible and where it is safe to do so. They will consider what adjustments in the home will make the home safe and/or not prejudicial to the child's/adolescent's health. This may include, for example, arrangements for a potentially abusive father to live elsewhere temporarily (where this can be robustly monitored) or for a younger child to live elsewhere out of harm's way from a volatile or disinhibited older mentally ill brother or sister. Grandparents are often willing to help out.

The family may of course themselves choose for their child to live elsewhere in a crisis or to relieve the crisis (e.g. with another family member), but if there are child protection concerns or it is felt that the family, in their private arrangements, are not taking the child's or adolescent's safety and well-being seriously, the duty social worker should be consulted.

Social and specialist housing

Social Services will sometimes find accommodation for young people under 16 with mental health problems, especially where these are socially determined. For under 16s, emergency placements are likely to be a choice

> **Box 10.1 Accommodation options for children and adolescents**
>
> - Home (with or without addition support or adjustment)
> - With other family or friends
> - Social care housing
>   - residential homes
>   - foster carer(s)
> - Homeless people's emergency housing
>   - hostels
>   - bed and breakfast
> - 'Supported accommodation' (semi-independent)
> - Specialist (high-intensity) supported accommodation

between an emergency foster placement, with a foster family prepared to offer a short-term home for the child or adolescent, especially for younger children, or a residential unit (a 'children's home'), where the young person will be supported by residential social workers working in shifts.

Even though Social Services children and families teams have social care responsibility for all young people 'in need' (including by virtue of mental illness) under 18, Social Services often do not have suitable accommodation within their usual placement options for an adolescent of 16 or over who has mental health difficulties or may have risks that appear to emanate from emotional difficulties (e.g. with a young person who self-harms repeatedly). Most Social Services will not place a 16- or 17-year-old in foster care unless there are very special circumstances or perhaps where they have been with that family before. 'Supported accommodation' options available to most Social Services child and family departments are usually designed to meet the needs of over-16s already in the care system, whose needs are primarily social and not further complicated by major mental health problems. However, that Social Services does not have (entirely) suitable residential or specialist foster-care placements for children and adolescents with mental health problems, who cannot live at home or at least have no stable home placement, does not absolve Social Services of their duty to support and protect, and accommodate such vulnerable young people. They may be required to organise and fund accommodation for young people via private social care agencies, with intensive supervision and support. This is unlikely to be available in an emergency (usually these funding arrangements are made by joint agency panels which most commonly meet at monthly intervals).

For 16- and 17-year-olds, there are usually meagre resources, if anything at all, other than bed and breakfast accommodation or hostels for homeless adolescents, and very little to support them once placed (inadequately) by housing departments.

Once young people turn 18, they become entitled to a variety of mental health 'supported housing' arrangements within the Supported Living scheme, with various levels of support according to need. Mental health-supported housing for 18-year-olds and over is funded, via the Supporting People programme (www.spkweb.org.uk), by a central grant administered through mental health housing panels, whereby the housing is paid by housing benefit, and the social care component comes out of a pooled Social Services and mental health budget, with a commitment from Social Services (adult) mental health team social workers (within community mental health teams) to support these vulnerable people. Paradoxically there is no such organised financial housing and social care support available for 16- and 17-year-olds, even though they are theoretically more vulnerable. The Supporting People arrangements should apply to adolescents of 16 or over, although the funding stream for specialist mental health supported housing is not clear.

Legal framework

Social workers may help to place children or adolescents without a formalised statutory contract, but it would be more usual for the social worker to 'accommodate' the young person with the collaboration of the parent(s) under Section 20 of the Children Act 1989. Parental responsibility in that case remains with the parent(s). In an emergency, if the child needs protection and the parent is not taking appropriate responsibility for the child's safety and welfare, or indeed is exaggerating the risk to the child, the professional involved may take out an emergency protection order to allow them to place the child in a place of safety.

Services for 16- and 17-year-olds

Commissioners should ensure that agreements are in place between paediatric, CAMHS and adult mental health services for the assessment and treatment of 16- and 17-year-olds, including agreeing thresholds for admission and the provision of suitable designated beds if they need admission.

If they are to be admitted to an adult mental health bed, written arrangements for this to happen in a way that best protects the young person from abuse and humiliation should be in place. This should include advice on dealing with the young person's and the family's understandable fears and misgivings. The preferred arrangement would be for the young person to be nursed in a single room with 1:1 nursing by nurses who have been checked by the Criminal Records Bureau (CRB), and who have access to advice from a CAMHS nurse (preferably) or another suitable CAMHS professional. The young person should be transferred to a designated adolescent unit bed at the earliest opportunity (see also Department of Health, 2004).

There should be a written protocol for carrying out Mental Health Act assessments on young people under 18. It would be good practice for at least one doctor to be trained in child and adolescent psychiatry (consultant,

117

specialist registrar or suitably experienced and trained staff grade doctor). Since the move to specialisation in social work, there are very few social workers who are both approved under the Mental Health Act, and child and family trained. In some areas, a Mental Health Act assessment will involve both the approved social worker and a social worker from the child and family department of Social Services.

Frequent attenders[1]

With regard to children, it is usually the parent who presents the child with a frequency that is thought to be excessive. The parent is perceived (and often disparaged) as 'over-anxious', and the child's distress may be minimised by staff. In the adult population at least, frequent attenders have a high degree of comorbidity and physical complaints should not be assumed automatically to be 'somatisation'. Young people who repeatedly self-harm may attend frequently for medical attention, or to get emotional support from professionals or to engage others in their support network (see also Chapter 5).

Why do they present frequently?

Often in these cases, the surface/presenting problem is attended to (albeit cursorily in most cases), but the underlying problems go on unresolved, leading to further emergency attendances, and inconsistent and fragmented healthcare.

Staff untrained to understand and deal with this under- or disorganised and dependent, reassurance-seeking group of service users may be prone to frustration with and denigration of such help-seekers, whose reactions to their problems seem exaggerated, their coping ability less than could be expected and who increase waiting times for other, 'more deserving' patients. However, the professional's consequent rejecting tone can amplify the user's need to be taken seriously and lead to an escalation of care-seeking behaviour. With parents anxious about their child's distress, minimising or dismissing the child's complaints may fuel the parent's worry that something important is being overlooked and lead to behaviour towards staff that then 'confirms' that they are unreasonable and 'over-anxious' parents, or even that the parents are encouraging illness behaviour in the child for the parent's gratification. (Of course, factitious illness and child neglect must also be considered where appropriate.)

In the adult population, frequent attenders are frequent users of healthcare in general and tend to have multiple complex problems including physical and psychological illness, cognitive impairment, psychosocial difficulties, and alcohol and substance misuse. These factors may apply

---

1. This and subsequent sections have been adapted from Royal College of Psychiatrists (2004a).

also to the parents of frequently attending children, but also to some older adolescents, especially in those whom vulnerability is increased by homelessness or unsupported, inappropriate housing and social isolation. Often these already vulnerable people have not and/or will not engage with primary care and Social Services, thus compounding their difficulties.

Effectively dealing with frequent attenders

- Frequent attendance should be considered an explicit clinical problem.
- Patients/parents with ill children who frequently attend should be identified and background information obtained from other healthcare providers.
- Multidisciplinary, multi-agency, across mental healthcare trust review of the frequent user should guide management.
- Individual guidelines for future management should include: typical presentation; past medical and psychiatric history; social history (and any involvement of Social Services, especially any child protection concerns); agreements/suggestions for future care (including a 'crisis plan'); and contact details of the professionals involved in providing care. (This may be done according to the care programme approach for appropriately identified young people or adults with mental health needs who have young children.)
- The 'patient's passport' (or 'Green card'), allowing the patient direct access to a ward and ward staff team used to dealing with them, has been found to be useful in some centres and with some identified patients.
- Patients who do not have a GP should be encouraged to register with one and be given the necessary information to facilitate this.
- Emergency department staff should have training to assist in the recognition of somatisation, psychiatric comorbidity and substance misuse.
- All staff in the emergency department should be trained to deal with patients (including the parents of sick children) who present with demanding and challenging behaviour. This should include recognising and dealing with the feelings evoked by such patients.

Patients who do not wait to be seen

Most young people who present themselves to the emergency department with mental health-related problems and then do not wait to be seen are intoxicated and/or have self-harmed. Classically, they leave without providing reassurance that they will be OK and will take proper responsibility for their safety. Emergency department staff are left worrying about their further risk of deliberate or accidental injury.

Detecting that the patient may not wait to be seen is or should be an important aspect of triage, especially if the person appears agitated. If the risk assessment suggests that the young person is at risk of self-harm (or further self-harm) and at risk of absconding, strenuous effort should be made to ensure that the young person does not leave or take their own discharge – this may include consideration of the use of common law duty to protect, or compulsory detention under the Mental Health Act Section 5.4 (a nurse's holding powers – for up to 4h) or Section 5.2 (a doctor's holding powers – for up to 72h).

- The patient's appearance should be carefully recorded to facilitate search and recovery by the police or hospital security staff, should the patient abscond.
- The patient should be monitored closely and with sensitivity, with staff providing support and comfort, and not just surveillance – where risks are high, one-to-one supportive supervision should be provided by an appropriate member of staff.
- Their being seen, assessed and treated should be prioritised.
- They should be kept informed of waiting time and what is being done to expedite their assessment.
- If truculent or resistive, they should be told explicitly what their rights are and what your duty and your department's policy is, should they leave before they are attended to and a risk assessment made.

The patient who has left before being seen

If a child/adolescent at risk of self-harming leaves before they are properly assessed, staff should err on the side of caution and:

- assume that they are at high risk, unless there are clear indicators that they are not;
- make every effort to contact them, if any contact details are available;
- alert hospital security, as they may still be in the hospital grounds, perhaps vacillating about whether to get help or not;
- contact the young person's parent(s)/carer(s) – it is permissible to contact them without the patient's permission in order to protect and safeguard them;
- inform the police, and specify the degree of risk – if the young person's whereabouts are known, the police should be invited to escort the person back for assessment, if necessary using statutory powers under Section 135 or 136 of the Mental Health Act 1983 (in England and Wales, and the equivalent powers in other jurisdictions).

Child abuse

Child abuse should be considered when a parent, bringing a young child to the emergency department, leaves without warning. This sudden departure may be considered a dereliction of parental responsibility (i.e. neglect) – the parent does not get the child the medical care they requires, or may be the result of the parent's anxiety that previous child abuse will be uncovered by the staff checking the child protection register.

CHAPTER 11

Confidentiality and information sharing

Tony Kaplan and Tricia Brennan

Principles of confidentiality and sharing information

Children and adolescents (or their parents) will, in the context of your assessment, trust you with information that they regard as private and sensitive. Children and adolescents have the same right to confidentiality as an adult. Knowing that their discussion with you is in confidence may allow them to talk about things in a more open and honest, and in a less inhibited and self-censoring way. This is of course clinically valuable and permits a better understanding of their anxieties and dilemmas, and helps to establish the therapeutic relationship. Many, however, will be impeded by their worry about the possibility of confidentiality being breeched – that your divulging this information to certain others would cause hurt or trouble to them or to others, and might lead to punishment, victimisation, shame and humiliation.

While reassuring patients and their parents about the obligation to preserve doctor–patient confidentiality, you should be clear about the limits of confidentiality and when you might be required to breech these limits in the patient's interest or where required to by law. This is good practice and respectful of the trust the patient places in you. The National Health Service (NHS) Code of Practice on confidentiality (Department of Health, 2003a) advises that patients are made aware that information about their clinical assessment and care will be shared only within the clinical team dealing directly with their immediate health problem. This is essential for optimum treatment and care. The patient, if they object to even this disclosure, should be made aware of the implications of this restriction of information for their care and treatment. Ultimately, however, their wishes must be respected, unless the practitioner is prepared to justify disclosure against the wishes of the patient 'in the public interest' and/or to prevent serious harm (to the patient or others).

The General Medical Council (2004), in their brief guidance, identify three guiding principles for disclosure of confidential information:

- wherever possible, patient's consent should be obtained before information is disclosed to others;
- disclosure should be kept to a minimum (on a 'need to know' basis);
- disclosure must be 'justifiable' – that the benefits to the patient and to the public outweigh the harm (to the patient, and to the trusting relationship between the patient and the doctor and medical services in general). The reasons for disclosure against the patient's wishes or without their consent or knowledge must be recorded in their case notes.

Sharing information a child/adolescent has given you in confidence with their parent, or sharing information the parent has divulged with the child/adolescent, may be tricky and require sensitivity and diplomacy. If, following your assessment, you determine that the young patient is incapable of giving consent to treatment or disclosure (see Chapter 7) because of immaturity, illness or incapacity, you may, according to the General Medical Council, disclose information to the relevant person or authority if you consider this to be in their medical interest. However, even when the young person is regarded as incapacitous, you should try to persuade them to give consent to the disclosure or at least allow an appropriate person they trust to be involved in the decision to disclose information.

Confidentiality and self-harm/risk-taking behaviour

This dilemma commonly arises when a young person has self-harmed (e.g. suicidal behaviour, maladaptive coping behaviour or as part of an eating disorder), or has indulged in extreme risk-taking behaviour (related to drugs, alcohol, casual sex or thrill-seeking). They may ask you not to tell their parents/carers.

There are two overriding principles involved in deciding whether to breech confidentiality or not.

If the young person is under 16 and/or not competent/capacitous, those with parental responsibility have a right to have information about any serious injury (or illness) the young person has suffered, so that they can exercise their parental responsibility in dealing with professionals to provide their child with what they regard as the best and most appropriate services available.

If the young person is over 16 and/or competent/capacitous, information about their self-harming or self-destructive behaviour must nevertheless be shared with anyone vital to the making of a robust risk-management plan, including the parents/carers (if this applies to them) – the justification for disclosure is the prevention of (further) significant harm.

As indicated above, you should always try to obtain consent from the patient, and you must explain and record any decision to disclose against their wishes.

Confidentiality and safeguarding children

Staff often need to share information about a patient with other health staff and staff from other agencies such as Social Services for the purpose of safeguarding and promoting the welfare of the child or adolescent. In cases where there may be child protection concerns, the information from a range of sources needs to be put together to establish whether the child is seen to be in need or at risk of harm.

Although health staff accept that they share patient information within a healthcare team, staff in general and doctors in particular are anxious about the legal and ethical restrictions on sharing information with other agencies. You should be aware of the law and of guidance applicable to the profession (Department of Health 2003b; Royal College of Paediatrics and Child Health, 2004). There is rarely an absolute barrier for the exchange of information, but the information given must be proportionate – a proportionate response to the need to protect the welfare of a child to whom the confidential information relates.

If there are concerns about the welfare and safety of a child, staff should inform Social Services about the concerns. Ideally, the child's/adolescent's and the parent's consent should be sought to share the information, and if given, there should be no problem. If consent is denied, then you should discuss the case with a senior colleague or designated professional such as the designated doctor for child protection in your area. You need to decide whether the circumstances justify the disclosure, taking into account what is being disclosed, for what purposes and to whom.

Several areas of the law impact on disclosure of information where a child may be at risk of harm.

Common duty of law

A duty of confidence exists where a contract provides information that should be kept confidential, and the special relationship between patient and doctor is one such contract. However, the duty is not absolute and can be justified if:

- the information is not confidential;
- the person to whom it is owed has authorised the disclosure;
- there is an overriding public interest in disclosure – the law recognises that this includes the public interest to prevent harm to others;
- disclosure is required by a court order or other legal obligation.

If information is disclosed to protect the welfare of the child, you should consider the proportionality of the information to be disclosed – that the amount of information and the number of people to whom it should be disclosed should only be that which is strictly necessary for the purpose of protecting the child. Only disclose information on a need-to-know basis.

Human Rights Act 1998

Article 8 of the European Convention on Human Rights (which forms part of UK law under the Human Rights Act 1998) recognises a right to respect for private and family life. However, the right is not absolute and disclosure of confidential information to protect the welfare of a child may be justified if it is necessary to prevent crime or to protect the health and welfare of a child. The same proportionality test applies as in common law.

Data Protection Act 1998

The Data Protection Act 1998 regulates the handling of personal information data and lays down requirements for obtaining, recording, storing and disclosing it. However, this should not be an obstacle if:

- you have particular concerns about the welfare of a child;
- you disclose information to Social Services or to another professional;
- the disclosure is justified under the common law duty of confidence.

Sections 17 and 47 of the Children Act 1989

The Children Act 1989 enables the Local Authority to request help from specified agencies, of which health is one, and places an obligation on those authorities to cooperate. This includes a request for information as part of a Section 47 (child protection) or a Section 17 (child in need) investigation.

Section 115 of the Crime and Disorder Act 1998

This act enables any person to disclose information to a relevant authority such as Local Authorities, NHS bodies and the police, for the prevention and reduction of crime and the identification or apprehension of offenders.

A Fraser (Gillick) competent child/adolescent may give consent themselves in the absence of parental consent. However, if a Fraser (Gillick) competent child refuses consent, a person with parental responsibility may consent to treatment or investigations in the child's best interests. If consent is denied by both competent child and parent, and if you have reasonable grounds to believe a child is at risk of significant harm, then the facts should still be reported to Social Services and the health staff should be prepared to take a role in the multi-agency assessment of a case.

Adult psychiatrists, GPs and other staff who look after adults who are parents may identify an illness/problem in the parent (e.g. alcoholism) that could impact on the ability to properly parent a child. If they have concerns about the welfare of the child, then the parent's doctor must refer the family to Social Services.

The General Medical Council's (2004) advice to doctors is:

'If you believe a patient to be a victim of neglect or physical, sexual or emotional abuse and that the patient cannot give or withhold consent to disclosure, you must give information promptly to an appropriate, responsible person or statutory agency, where you believe that the disclosure is in the patient's best interests. If, for any reason, you believe that disclosure of information is not in the best interests of an abused or neglected patient, you should discuss the issues with an experienced colleague. If you decide not to disclose information, you must be prepared to justify your decision.'

CHAPTER 12

Practitioners and pathways: a competency framework

Tony Kaplan, Paul Gill, Diana Hulbert, Avril Washington, Ian Maconochie and Annie Souter

Not all children who are assessed in the emergency department present to the department directly. They are referred to the 'acute service', which for children is the emergency department and paediatrics combined (Fig. 12.1). Paediatric consultants who run hotline services will have often taken referrals from GPs, schools amd Social Services. Where that service is not available, paediatric specialist registrars will take referrals. They will usually elect to assess the patient in the emergency department, but the referral is to the service rather than to the emergency department *per se*.

Because service organisation and resources vary so greatly from place to place, this chapter will be presented according to the place along the referral pathway from community to in-patient services where different organisations of professionals operate. The pathways vary from hospital to hospital and so cannot be specified. Thus, a number of 'access points' (or assessment and treatment points) will be demarcated. At each of these, the role and function of the professionals involved will be clarified.

The competencies (knowledge and skills base) for professional staff at each access point (from whichever discipline or grade) (Box 12.1) are made up of competencies that are assumed for all first-line doctors and specialist nurses (see *Common competencies for doctors and nurses*, pp. 127–129), and specialist competencies related to their particular role and function (elucidated for each access point separately). These competencies pertain to making an assessment, to intervene therapeutically if possible and to make a useful and effective referral on (and/or to take a referral). Although practitioners will share the 'common competencies' in their breadth, specialists will naturally be assumed to have greater in-depth competency in their specialist domain, separately, and as these apply to the common competencies. For example, conducting a mental state examination – establishing and describing how the child or adolescent is thinking and feeling – is regarded as a common competency, but a mental health practitioner is expected to be able to do a more thorough examination of the young person's mental state, especially with regard to unusual mental states, and the CAMHS professional is expected to be even more in tune with establishing a younger child's state of mind.

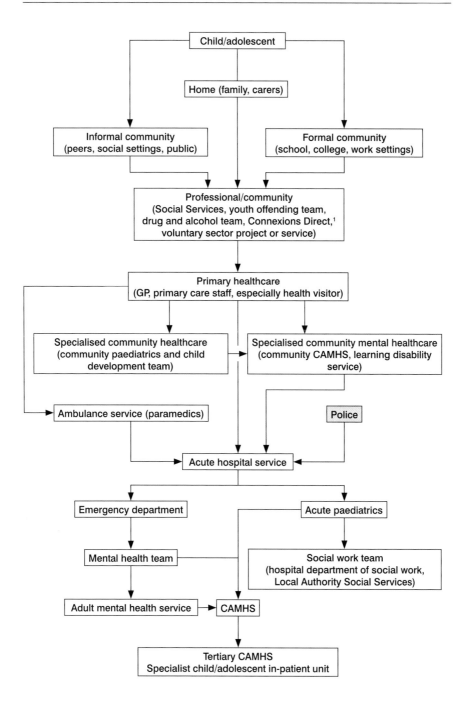

Fig. 12.1 Care pathway. CAMHS, child and adolescent mental health service; GP, general practitioner.

1. Service offering help and advice for 13- to 19-year-olds (www.connexions-direct.com).

Box 12.1 Staff at each access point along the care pathway

- Primary care and community CAMHS
- Paramedic/ambulance staff
- Emergency department generic staff/triage
- Paediatric first-line staff
- Psychiatric first-line staff
- CAMHS first-line (or on-call) staff
- Social Services first-line staff (the duty social worker/approved social worker)

A pro forma for referral is included below. Making useful referrals on is a common competency, as is taking a referral in a calm, thoughtful and respectful way. Effective communication between professionals and good team work in the emergency department is essential in helping children, adolescents and their families in crisis.

Trainers and teachers may wish to match their trainees or juniors against these standards to identify their training needs. This book will be a useful resource to help practitioners meet their training needs.

The good practice guidelines defined by the National Insitute for Mental Health in England (2006a) (Appendix IV) are endorsed and presumed to underpin the practice of all staff (Box 12.1), whether they are designated as mental health staff or not.

Common competencies for doctors and nurses

- To be able to take a referral of a child or adolescent in a calm, thoughtful and organised way.
- To be able to engage a child or adolescent, separately and with their family: to talk to the child, adolescent and parents in a calm, sensitive and respectful manner, and to use age-appropriate language, to conduct the consultation in such a way that a child or adolescent and their family feel able to talk about difficult or emotional issues.
- To know enough about the legal framework as it relates to children and adolescents:

  - to understand parental responsibility, the scope and limits of the powers parents/guardians have to make decisions for the child and who by right needs to be involved in accessing further services;
  - to make a brief assessment of the young person's capacity and competence to give and withhold consent to treatment, and to be aware of the rights of 16- and 17-year-olds under the Mental Capacity Act;
  - to make decisions about the right to confidentiality and when to breech confidentiality in the patient's interest as required by the law;

- to understand the applicability of the Mental Health Act;
- to understand and follow the principle that the child's needs are paramount and that all decisions are to be made in the best interests of the child or adolescent in their care.

- To be able to take a history accurately and sensitively, and to record accurately, fully and legibly the nature of the problem, including contributory, aggravating and ameliorating factors in causation and maintenance that routinely includes biological, psychological, educational and social factors; to understand the young person's family and social circumstances and how these may influence outcome; and to understand how the young person copes with adversity, specifically with the kind of adversity that has led to the current crisis.
- To do an initial assessment of and to know the signs and symptoms that indicate mental health presentation in a child or adolescent, including serious conditions such as depression, psychosis, ADHD and autism-spectrum disorders.
- To be able to conduct a mental state examination.
- To do an assessment of risk to self and others, most importantly to know the common risk and protective factors for suicide and self-harm in young people, and to evaluate this alongside the risks suggested by circumstantial factors and the mental state examination.
- To know about the management of common causes of admission to hospital owing to psychological distress such as self-harm, according to your role and responsibility.
- To know the child protection policies and procedures as locally agreed.
- To work with colleagues in multidisciplinary teams to ensure consistency and continuity, and a holistic approach to the treatment and care of children and adolescents.
- To know and acknowledge the limits of your competence and to know when to ask for help, support and supervision, and to know who to consult.
- To be able to make an informed referral on, to have an appreciation of which patients must be directly referred to a another team/agency/ward, and to know which team/agency/ward to refer to appropriately according to the protocols agreed between the emergency department, the paediatric department and the mental health teams (Box 12.2).

Roles, functions and specific competencies

Primary care staff (and community CAMHS)

Role

- Where possible and practical, to assess and treat emotional and behavioural (mental health) problems in the community.

Box 12.2. Essential information for making a referral

- Time and date of referral
- Name and contact details of referrer
- Name of patient
- Date of birth/age of patient
- Address of patient
- Who has parental responsibility/next of kin?
- GP
- Other professionals/agencies involved (and why)
  - known to CAMHS?
  - known to the emergency department?
  - known to Social Services? On the child protection register?
- Presenting problem
  - family and social circumstances
  - relevant previous history
- Current mental state
- Risk assessment
  - known risks
  - risks as assessed
  - factors increasing or reducing risk
  - risk management interventions and plans to limit/contain/reduce risk
- What can't be managed in the current setting that required further intervention/admission?
- Desired outcome from referral

- To make an informed referral on to hospital services where the problems cannot be managed in the community.

Function

- To understand the nature of the problem.
- To determine that the risk of continuing significant disturbance/disorder or of serious deterioration cannot be managed safely other than by referral to the emergency department (or acute hospital services).
- To establish that suffering cannot be ameliorated effectively and reliably other than by referral to the emergency department (or acute hospital services).
- Or, that urgent treatment is required and that treatment can only happen properly in a hospital setting, and/or that hospital admission is likely to be necessary to carry out the treatment.

Specific competencies (in addition to the common competencies)

- To know enough about the presentation and complications of mental health problems in children and adolescents to determine that further/emergency assessment in a hospital setting is relevant and warranted, and that health services are likely to be the agencies that are most able to contribute to the solution of the crisis.

- To access already available information and past history within that primary care (or CAMHS) setting, make clinical judgements of relevance and summarising this in the referral on.
- To know what local services, other than the emergency department, could provide immediate support, advice and/or interventions or be available to provide a timely assessment so as to obviate the need for an emergency referral to the emergency department, and how to access these.

Paramedic and ambulance staff

Role

- To offer emergency medical treatment where necessary.
- To transport the patient safely to hospital if indicated.

Function

In addition to all the functions of primary care staff (p.129) in determining that admission to an acute hospital service/emergency department is required:

- to understand the nature of the problem requiring the calling out of an emergency vehicle and crew;
- to provide first aid treatment or secondary prevention in cases of self-harm;
- to ensure the safety of the patient;
- to access necessary information to intervene effectively according to the context;
- to transport the patient to the emergency department as necessary in as timely, safe and comfortable way as possible;
- to gather information at the scene to aid further assessment.

Specific competencies (in addition to the common competencies)

- To be able to offer emergency/first aid treatment for self-harm as per the NICE (2004) guidelines.

Emergency department staff

For doctors in the emergency department, these are the competencies agreed with the College of Emergency Medicine. These are the things your senior colleagues expect you to know and know how to do. It is presumed that if practitioners from other disciplines, especially nurses, because of local service configuration are required to carry the same responsibility as doctors, they will have equivalent competencies. If there are things listed below that you feel you don't know or know how to do, look elsewhere in the book for guidance or raise this with your head of department as a training issue.

Role

- To assess quickly to determine the degree of urgency required for intervention.
- To ensure that the patient is safe and that their wait for treatment does not incur unnecessary distress or suffering.
- To offer timely intervention within the competence of the emergency department practitioner.
- To determine whether the problem will require the intervention of a specialist and then to refer on.

Specific competencies (in addition to the common competencies)

Competencies appropriate to all emergency department staff

- To be able to recognise the degree of urgency of the patient's needs.
- To be able to evaluate the degree of danger the patient poses to self and/or others.
- To be able to make a brief risk assessment for self-harm based on a knowledge of indicators of risk.
- To be able to employ de-escalation techniques in emotionally charged situations.
- To know the protocols for those patients who leave before assessment and/or treatment.
- To know that child protection issues have to be taken into consideration in all cases of children and adolescents attending the emergency department, whether as index patients or when accompanying parents who are physically or mentally ill.

Reception staff

- To be able to listen to the patient and their carers, and intervene in a calm, non-threatening way.

Triage staff

- To take a time-efficient, focused history from child and adolescent patients and their carers, with a recognition that taking a history from both is necessary.
- To be able to make an initial risk assessment (and to have the clinical 'tools' for this; see for example Appendix VI), and to make an initial risk assessment plan.

Departmental doctors and nurse specialists

- To be able to take a history, conduct an examination and do the necessary preliminary investigations sufficient to rule out an organic contribution to the presenting problem.

Senior staff

- To have an in-depth knowledge of the organic conditions that can present as acute mental health problems in children and adolescents.

- To have a detailed understanding of capacity, consent issues as applied to children and adolescents, the Mental Health Act and its applications, the scope of and availability of community support, and other discharge planning issues.
- To be able and willing to discuss difficult cases with other senior colleagues from other specialist departments and disciplines in an informed way to arrive at the best plan for intervention, including the decision that in the particular case waiting longer than the 4h mandatory waiting limit must be contravened in the patient's best interest.

The curriculum for emergency medicine includes the specific paediatric objectives in psychiatry as follows.

- Understand normal behaviour patterns including response to injury and illness from birth to adolescence.
- Be able to recognise abnormal child behaviour patterns.
- Understand the influence of physical, emotional and social factors on development and health.
- Understand excessive crying, its causes and the resources available to help families.
- Understand the roles of other professions, agencies and the voluntary sector.
- Understand the emotional impact of hospitalisation on children.
- Be able to recognise fabricated illness and injury in children.
- Understand adolescent behaviour in maturation.
- Be able to recognise and refer patients presenting with self-harm.
- Understand the multidisciplinary nature of CAMHS.
- Understand the signs and symptoms that indicate serious conditions such as depression and psychosis.

Paediatric and first-line staff

For paediatric doctors (in training), these are the competencies that have been agreed with your Royal College. These are the things your senior colleagues expect you to know and know how to do. For specialist nurses to carry the same responsibility, they should have equivalent competencies in assessment. If there are items listed below that you feel you don't know or know how to do, look elsewhere in the book for guidance or raise this with your head of department as a training issue.

Role

- To assess all children and adolescents referred (up to the age of 16, or up to the age of 18 depending on local agreements and arangements; see also *Adult mental health first-line staff*, p. 135) whatever their perceived problem, and make informed decisions as to the need for and type of intervention, including the need to refer on.

Function

Paediatric junior staff should take a sufficiently detailed history, conduct an appropriate examination and undertake any investigations required in order to:

- assess the relative contributions of physical and/or mental ill health to the presentation;
- make a preliminary assessment of the risk that the patient presents to themselves, their family, other patients and to staff;
- gauge the severity of the problem;
- decide whether discharge with or without a mental health referral, admission to a paediatric ward and mental health assessment the following day, or a more urgent assessment is appropriate;
- determine the child's/adolescent's need for protection, and liaise with Social Services appropriately.

If more urgent assessment is thought to be appropriate, then the child/adolescent should be discussed with the paediatric consultant on call/paediatric emergency department consultant in order to:

- determine whether an urgent assessment is appropriate, and if so to follow locally agreed protocols as to who should be contacted, the timing and location of the assessment;
- to ensure the safety and ongoing medical care of the young person while waiting for that assessment;
- to participate in discussions about placement of the young person once the assessment is complete, considering the safety of the patient and others, and the level of supervision that may be required.

Specific competencies (in addition to the common competencies)

- To have begun to develop skills in the management of emotionally complex family situations.
- To understand the duties and responsibilities of a paediatrician in the safeguarding of all children and adolescents.
- To be familiar with local and national clinical guidelines and protocols in paediatric practice.

CAMHS first-line staff

Role

The role of first-line CAMHS staff in the emergency department depends on local service arrangements and agreements. Some centres will have a CAMHS liaison team to address CAMHS emergencies, at least during working hours. Some will have CAMHS doctors in training available to intervene directly, but often (paradoxically) out of hours only. Most have CAMHS senior professionals offering consultation on the telephone and available to carry out a specialist assessment the next working day.

Function

- With regard to children and adolescents under 16, to consult with paediatric first-line staff and to provide advice on their emergency management.
- With regard to young people of 16 and 17, to consult with adult mental health first-line staff and to provide advice on their emergency management.
- Where consultation is insufficient to resolve the problems presented, and where resources permit, to contribute to the assessment and emergency intervention and management directly.
- To contribute to the referral on to a specialist in-patient mental health unit if required (if no other disposal is available that would ensure the patient's safety and protect against serious deterioration in their condition until they could be seen by a suitable qualified CAMHS professional).
- To offer an assessment directly, if the patient is admitted, on the next working day.

Specific competencies (in addition to the common competencies)

- To have sufficient skills in consulting with other professionals, especially understanding the problems that the professional needs to resolve, and through a process of systematic questioning, helping to reach a set of conclusions about the best way forward.
- To be able to take a full developmental history, understanding the implications and predictive value of early events, attainments, difficulties and relationships in the child's life.
- To have a specialist knowledge about child and adolescent mental health and behavioural problems and their presentations, including the alerting signs and symptoms of child abuse.
- To have sufficient therapeutic skills to provide crisis intervention.
- To develop a risk management plan in consultation with other professionals if necessary, including other (senior) CAMHS colleagues, which may include referring on for urgent admission to a specialist Tier 4 adolescent in-patient unit or to a CAMHS community team for out-patient follow-up.
- To know how to manage a difficult (16- or 17-year-old) patient, including being able to prescribe rapid tranquillisation.
- To be involved in considering the use of the Children Act or the relevant Mental Health Act to detain a young person in hospital against their wishes if so indicated by the risk management plan.
- To know where to refer on to and how, and what funding arrangements are in place for specialist in-patient mental health units.
- To have knowledge of local resources relevant to the need of children and adolescents with mental health crises.
- To contribute to establishing that the young person's needs for protection and care are met on an adult mental health ward, if the patient is admitted there because no other suitable placement is available.

Adult mental health first-line staff

Role

The role of first-line adult mental health staff in assessing children and adolescents with mental health problems in the emergency department will depend on local arrangements and agreements. Rarely, paediatrics will assume responsibility for the initial assessment of all young people up to 18 (as required by the NSF for children, young people and maternity services; Department of Health, 2004). It is more usual for 16- and 17-year-olds with perceived mental health problems to be seen in the first instance by a member of the adult mental health team. In some hospitals the crisis team will see all new cases in the emergency department of 16- and 17-year-olds. In others where there is an adult liaison team available (often only during normal working hours), they will see this population. However, most commonly, the junior doctor on call for psychiatry (or increasingly, the specialist nurse practitioner) will do the initial assessment on this age group, sometimes in consultation with a CAMHS professional on call. Very occasionally, adult mental health first-line staff will be called by the paediatrician to offer advice, assessment or intervention with a very acutely disturbed child under 16 where no emergency CAMHS is available, or where the CAMHS senior doctor is available only for telephone consultation, or it is the agreement that they provide telephone consultation only unless their attendance is imperative.

Function

For children under 16 years

- To consult with the paediatric team in an emergency situation (where local resources allow for a CAMHS consultant or specialist registrar on call on the telephone only), especially with regard to understanding abnormal mental states, usually in consultation with a CAMHS professional on call – this will normally include contributing to an enhanced risk assessment, taking into account known risk indicators, circumstantial factors and the mental state examination. This may require conducting a mental state examination (on adolescents almost exclusively), only where essential for risk management.

For 16- and 17-year-olds

- To make an assessment of their emergency mental health needs and to intervene accordingly, usually in consultation with a CAMHS professional on call – this will include a risk assessment and risk management plan.

For all children and adolescents: to be involved in considering the application of the Mental Health Act.

Competencies

The competencies for adult psychiatrists and trainees, and for mental health nurse specialist practitioners, are the common competencies listed earlier, and are essentially the same as for child mental health professionals working in this domain, in breadth if not in depth. The competencies detailed earlier for CAMHS are assumed to apply also to adult mental health first-line staff (or junior doctors at least), although of course CAMHS staff will have more detailed knowledge in their specialist area (e.g. in relation to child-specific syndromes and local children's resources). Adult mental health professionals should be able to interview children and adolescents sufficiently well to conduct a brief mental state examination (with enough detail to discuss it fully with a CAMHS colleague on call, who may be able to help to contextualise the findings in terms of the child's development and family and social system) and to be sufficiently flexible in approach, so that skills and knowledge gained in managing adults are adapted to the context of younger people and not simply transposed. The adult mental health practitioner is expected to be more knowledgeable about and familiar with the Mental Health Act (compared with the CAMHS professional) and will have a special role in establishing a safe environment if an adolescent is admitted to an adult mental health ward (pp. 150–151).

Social Services first-line staff

Role

To some extent, the role of the social worker in the emergency department is dependent on local service arrangements and agreements. In some hospitals, the social worker who will see the patient and family will be part of a CAMHS liaison team, and thus have extensive CAMHS experience, and their role and competencies will be those that apply to all CAMHS first-line workers (pp. 134–135). In some centres, the social worker will be part of an adult mental health liaison team, and their role and competencies will be those for other adult mental health first-line professionals. Where the social worker is a paediatric (hospital) social worker, especially where there is a paediatric emergency department, the generic competencies for all child and adolescent health service workers may apply, but the social worker in that situation will usually be involved because of their specialist skills and knowledge with regard to psychosocial enquiry and child protection. Especially out of hours, the social worker will be the duty social worker, who may or may not have much experience with children and families, but will be expected to know enough to fulfil the fundamental aspects of social work assessment with children, especially with regard to child protection and the scope of the relevant child legislation.

Although some social workers may be approved to conduct assessments under the relevant Mental Health Act, this is not reliably or even usually the case, and where a specialist mental health assessment is to be conducted by a social worker to consider compulsory detention under the Mental Health Act, an approved social worker, usually on rostered duty, will have to be called in. (In England and Wales, the Mental Health Act 1983 has been ammended, coming into force in 2008. The role of the approved social worker has been replaced by the role of the approved mental health practitioner, who may be a social worker; however, approved mental health practitioners could increasingly be drawn from other disciplines.) The approved social worker will be a specialist in mental health social work, and may have limited knowledge of and experience in applying child protection procedure. Child protection advice should always be obtained from a child and family social worker, or if necessary, in the first instance out of hours, from the duty social worker.

Function

In addition to the generic functions according to which team the social worker operates within, the social worker (other than the approved social worker/approved mental health professional) will be expected to do the following.

- To undertake any initial child protection risk assessment, paying attention to emotional/psychiatric issues, and to liaise with emergency department, paediatric, CAMHS and adult mental health staff on call with regard to subsequent management.
- To offer consultation to emergency department staff and paediatric staff on call, and agree assessment and management plans taking into account child protection procedures and provisions of the relevant Children Act operating in their jurisdiction.
- To advise on what Social Services' local (or in some cases, regional or even national) resources (e.g. emergency accommodation) may be required for the child/adolescent and their family to address the immediate crisis, including what relevant assessments need to be completed, and then what the referral and funding authorisation procedures are, including for specialist residential placements available to Social Services (or in some cases available only via multi-agency funding).
- To contribute to the risk assessment, taking social circumstances into account including, with regard to admission to a hospital ward, whether to a paediatric ward, especially whether the patient (and family) is (are) likely to be manageable/containable on the ward, or in the case of admission to an adult mental health ward, whether the patient will be safe from abuse or exploitation.
- To contribute to the multidisciplinary team assessment and emergency intervention.

Function of the approved social worker/approved mental health practitioner
- To make an assessment of the young person who is deemed to be at risk or to pose a significant risk to others as a consequence of mental disorder (or mental impairment), to determine that compulsory detention is the only way to ensure the patient's safety and the safety of others, and/or that the patient's health will suffer severely unless detained in hospital, and that there are no other solutions that will achieve the same purpose with less restriction of the patient's liberty.

Specific competencies

- The ability to make sound assessments of risk, with special reference to child protection.
- Skills in undertaking a 'social state' assessment, an holistic assessment, including a non-psychiatric 'mental state', which gives an indication of the global level of functioning in the patient and family and social networks. It will identify social and professional supports and strengths, and also identify any risk factors. This assessment will tell a 'story' of the child's/ adolescent's current state, significant past history and the events leading up to the presentation.
- To have a sound working knowledge of the relevant Children Act, child protection procedures and Mental Health Act operating in their jurisdiction.
- To know the rights and responsibilities under the Children Act of parents/carers of young people at risk.
- To know how to make and assessment of a young person's capacity to consent (or not) to treatment in differing situations, and where this might be overridden by a parent under the Children Act, or by the Inherent Jurisdiction of the court.
- To have knowledge of Local Authority resources, especially with regard to emergency placement/housing, relevant to the needs of children and adolescents with social and/or mental health crises and how to access these.

The interested reader is also referred to *The Social Work Contribution to Mental Health Services: The Future Direction* (National Institute for Mental Health in England, 2006).

Roles and responsibilities of senior staff

Child and adolescent psychiatry consultant

At a managerial level

- Advising governments, policy makers, the public sector authorities that are responsible for commissioning services and any public, independent, voluntary or private sector providers of healthcare who deliver services (including after- and longer-term care) for children and adolescents who present with mental health crises to the emergency department.
- Working with staff of child health and emergency departments and within other units that deliver services to develop, implement and monitor protocols for the psychosocial assessment and management of children and adolescents presenting to the emergency department in crisis. This should involve close liaison and cooperation between the medical, nursing and other relevant professional staff of specialist CAMH, adult mental health, paediatric, emergency, general medical, substance misuse and Social Services.

- Identifying the staffing levels and training required to provide comprehensive services for children and adolescents who are seen in the emergency department.
- Working with local commissioners and service providers to review implementation of this advice.

At an operational level

- Providing consultation and advice to relevant providers of acute care, emergency, paediatric and mental health services, appropriate to local need and within the context of comprehensive CAMHS.
- Advising on and being involved in delivering training for CAMHS staff and the staff of the paediatric, child health, emergency, social and education services departments in order to ensure that young people and their families and carers receive sufficient and appropriate immediate responses and aftercare relevant to their mental health crisis. In particular, this should involve involvement in developing and implementing modular programmes for training staff of primary healthcare, ambulance, emergency, paediatric and child health, and specialist child and adolescent mental health services in comprehensive psychosocial and risk assessment.
- Being available to teach and supervise junior medical staff and to consult with/to non-medical staff who are involved in assessing and managing children and adolescents who need emergency assessment and intervention as a consequence of a mental health crisis, including those who self-harm.
- In certain cases and circumstances, being involved directly in the direct clinical assessment of, intervention with and care of children and adolescents and their families or carers.

Paediatric consultant

At a managerial level

This may be delegated to the lead paediatrician for the emergency department or the lead paediatrician for CAMHS liaison but should be discussed with the whole consultant body.

- To participate fully in local planning of services for children presenting to the acute service with mental health problems. This may include attending the local emergency department paediatric liaison committee, liaising with the local CAMHS strategic partnership board and liaising with primary care.
- To ensure that robust local protocols exist for the management of children presenting to the hospital with acute mental health needs. These should be multidisciplinary, multi-agency agreements signed off by the senior officers of all organisations involved (e.g. acute trust, mental health trust, primary care trust and Local Authority).
- To ensure full implementation and audit of these protocols.

- To identify the training needs of the paediatric junior and senior staff with regard to children's mental heath issues and ensure appropriate training programmes are provided and attended, usually in liaison with local CAMHS professionals.

At an operational level

These roles and responsibilities apply to all consultant paediatricians who take part in the acute on-call service, whether in the daytime or out of hours.

- To be available to discuss any concerns colleagues in primary care, education services, Social Services, etc., may have about children presenting with possible acute mental health difficulties.
- To be able to give advice about local services that may be appropriate for children and adolescents if they do not need assessment in hospital.
- To coordinate the care of a child or adolescent presenting with an acute mental health problem.
- To ensure the medical aspects of any mental health presentation are dealt with appropriately and in a timely manner .
- To encourage junior staff to identify when they have reached the limit of their competence in managing a mental health or psychosocial difficulty and to respond promptly to a request for assistance.
- To assist junior staff directly in the management of emotionally complex families, of psychosocial difficulties requiring liaison with many agencies or disciplines, and of young people who are actively suicidal or acutely mentally ill.
- To undertake a preliminary mental state examination in order to determine if a mental health assessment is necessary and if so with what degree of urgency.
- To work sensitively in all dealings with the family in order to facilitate the referral to and hence engagement with mental health professionals and services.
- To have a working knowledge of the Children Act and sufficient knowledge of the Mental Health Act to be able to meet the needs of a child or adolescent with acute mental heath difficulties.
- To be familiar with legal and ethical frameworks about consent and confidentiality for this group of children and adolescents.
- To ensure that the placement of a young person who needs admission for an acute mental health problem is suitable for the young person and the family.
- To ensure adequate nursing numbers and support if the child or adolescent is to be admitted to a paediatric ward, including provision of specialist nursing if necessary.
- To consider any child protection concerns and involve Social Services as appropriate.
- To provide a debriefing opportunity, ideally in a multidisciplinary meeting, after the management of a particularly challenging case.

- To identify when local protocols have not worked and provide written feedback to the appropriate person.

Emergency department consultant

At a managerial level

- Advising governments, policy makers, the public sector authorities that are responsible for commissioning services, and any public, independent, voluntary or private sector providers of healthcare who deliver services for children and adolescents, and who may present with mental health needs to the emergency departments.
- Working with the staff from child health/paediatrics and CAMHS, and other units that deliver services to children and adolescents and their families to develop, implement and monitor protocols for the psychosocial assessment and management of children and adolescents who present to the emergency department. This should be multi-professional and include other relevant staff from adult mental health, general medicine, Social Services and substance misuse services.
- Identifying and lobbying for the staffing levels and training required to provide comprehensive services for children and adolescents with mental health problems who present to the emergency department.
- To establish regular meetings with the designated consultants, individually or within a liaison forum/committee.
- To ensure that there is good-quality training for the emergency department staff, including on child and adolescent mental health and child protection.
- To ensure that there is a robust child protection policy (in conjunction with the lead nurse for child protection).
- Ensuring that these recommendations are funded and met by the local commissioning agencies and service providers.

At an operational level

- Providing consultation and advice to the relevant providers of acute mental health and paediatric care within the trust and community;
- Advising on, and delivering the training in emergency medical management of this group of patients for staff from the emergency department, CAMHS, child health, Social Services and education staff. This should be at an appropriate level of detail to ensure the highest standards of care.
- Being available to teach and supervise junior medical staff and a resource for non-medical staff who are assessing and managing these children and adolescents who are presenting acutely to the service.
- Being available to see and assess particularly complex and problematic cases and being directly involved in their clinical care as a first or second opinion.

- To know, among other things, who is the named/designated consultant for adult mental health liaison and paediatric liaison (CAMHS liaison).
- To put in place protocols for commonly occurring conditions, including child and adolescent mental health presentations.
- To agree tools for psychosocial assessments.
- To have agreed referral protocols between departments and agencies.
- To have discharge protocols agreed with the departments and agencies required to deal with the case once discharged.
- To ensure that the routes for the use of the Mental Health Act are clear, and that the law and issues to do with consent and capacity/ competence under the Children Act, and issues of confidentiality with regard to children and adolescents are well understood by all the emergency department staff.

General adult/liaison consultant

At a managerial level

- Supporting CAMHS colleagues in providing consistent advice to policy-making bodies, commissioners and trust management.
- In collaboration with local CAMHS, the emergency department, and paediatric services, developing agreed care pathways for the management of young people attending the emergency department.
- To ensure that there is good-quality training for adult mental health professionals attending the emergency department, including on child and adolescent mental health and child protection.
- To establish regular meetings with the designated consultants, individually or within a liaison forum/committee and participating in it.

At an operational level

- Supervising junior medical staff and, where appropriate, staff from other disciplines.
- Ensuring that staff working in adult mental health services are aware of their limitations when involved in the care of young people.
- Being involved in the assessment and care of complex cases.
- To establish a working relationship with relevant CAMHS colleagues.
- To participate in relevant training for all disciplines.
- To establish evaluation procedures to ensure that agreed care pathways are followed, and that there are no major problems with those pathways.
- To ensure that there is a robust child protection policy (in conjunction with the lead nurse for child protection)
- To ensure that there is a clear procedure for following the relevant section of the Mental Health Act and that it is followed.

CHAPTER 13

Issues for department heads and managers

Tony Kaplan*

A number of agencies, disciplines and departments will (potentially) be required to make suitable arrangements to deal with children and adolescents with mental health-related problems who present in crisis to the hospital. These include primary care (who refer in), the police and the ambulance and paramedic service (who may bring the patient in), the emergency department, the adult mental health teams (assessment, duty and crisis intervention teams), the paediatric team, CAMHS (formal liaison team or *ad hoc*), Social Services (duty and hospital teams) and in some places voluntary sector services. These teams and agencies need to work together efficiently at their interfaces to ensure the smoothest and safest 'patient journey' through the system. They should have robust working arrangements and written agreements, protocols for cross-referral, good communication, management arrangements, including liaison committees, and clearly-demarcated responsibility for training and induction of junior staff, new staff, and agency and locum staff. This all needs to be jointly managed in an accountable way and audited, with mechanisms in place for feedback and change where necessary. Commissioners should ensure that a functioning service is in place to meet the needs of these children, adolescents and their families, and agree service standards in line with the NSF.

Management and liaison

The liaison committee

The NICE (2004) guidelines on self-harm and the Royal College of Psychiatrists (2004a, 2004b, 2006a) all recommend the establishment of an emergency department liaison committee. Where this has been implemented, it will be a local decision as to whether CAMHS and paediatric/child health services join this forum to discuss all cases presenting to the emergency

---

*With special thanks to Catherine Lavelle for her contribution (see p. vii).

department with mental health special needs whatever their age, or whether it would be more effective and appropriate for there to be a separate children and adolescent liaison committee. The latter may be more appropriate where there is a separate paediatric emergency department, as long as the needs of 16- and 17-year-olds are addressed. A CAMHS consultant should be nominated as having lead responsibility for liaising with the emergency department. The Royal College of Psychiatrists (2006a) recommends that a CAMHS consultant and a paediatric consultant take joint responsibility for setting up and chairing a paediatric liaison committee, and that may apply here – the liaison committee will in practice supersede any liaison committee overseeing policies and procedures regarding self-harm only.

Function

The agencies, disciplines and departments (potentially) involved, including primary care, the police, the ambulance service, the emergency department, adult mental health and CAMHS, paediatrics, Social Services and any relevant voluntary sector services, can in this forum:

- discuss and authorise robust working arrangements, written agreements and protocols for accepting and making (cross-) referrals;
- improve communication and develop a shared understanding of certain difficult presentations and their institutional responses;
- confirm management and administrative arrangements;
- agree responsibility for and plan training and induction of junior staff, new staff, agency and locum staff;
- agree standards and set up joint inter-departmental and inter-agency audit and evaluation cycles.

The paediatric liaison CAMHS team

The availability to the emergency departments of CAMHS around the country varies enormously in different areas and hospitals. Some hospitals have a specific paediatric liaison CAMHS team; others have some input from community CAMHS. It is recommended that all emergency departments should have access to on-call CAMHS.

Where a specific paediatric liaison mental health team exists within the hospital, the roles of that team include the following.

- Ensuring the emergency department staff and the paediatric team are aware of how to contact the on-call CAMHS.
- Working with the emergency department and paediatric teams to draw up protocols relevant to that hospital. Examples are protocols for the management of alcohol intoxication and of self-harm in young people (Appendix V).
- Contributing to training of medical, nursing and other staff in the emergency department (and paediatrics) on the protocols and on mental health issues in children and adolescents.

- Contributing to audits concerning child and adolescent mental health, paediatrics and the emergency department (e.g. audit of management of self-harm).
- Involvement, with the paediatric team in the identification and analysis of risk and serious incidents concerning children, adolescents and their families in the emergency department who present with mental health problems.
- Overall, the paediatric liaison team should ensure there is a clear line of communication between CAMHS, paediatrics and the emergency department. Ideally, the emergency department and paediatrics should identify one or more people to take an interest in child and adolescent mental health and to be involved, on behalf of the department, in drawing up protocols.

Interfacing between departments and agencies

Working with the police

Place of safety

The policy for children needs to be congruent with local agreements regarding designated 'places of safety' for adults, agreed with the local police force and covering the area of the local police force. Whether the emergency department is suitable as a designated place of safety for adolescents who may be violent is something that needs to be agreed locally according to resources. Paediatric staff may be well placed to provide de-escalation because they are usually more used to talking to upset adolescents than their adult colleagues, but issues of security/safety of staff and other children need to be considered.

There needs to be a written policy for each emergency department agreed locally between the emergency department, paediatrics, CAMHS, adult/general psychiatry, Social Services and the police. It is advisable for the following to form part of the agreement.

- The police agree to wait to provide assistance in the event of violence, and will wait until the matter is resolved, and if necessary, once the assessment has been completed satisfactorily, be prepared to remove the young person (and their family) from the emergency department if they do not require urgent medical treatment.
- Arrangements for the provision of a suitably trained responsible adult if the child/adolescent is to be interviewed by the police and is unaccompanied.
- Arrangements for the provision of emergency assessment of disturbed adolescents in police custody if they are so violent that they cannot be managed safely in the emergency department. The assessors need to be medically trained to make a brief assessment as to whether the patient may be in the throes of an organic confusional state, and be

able to access advise on appropriate sedation that will allow a fuller assessment safely in a medical setting.

- Arrangements for assessments of young people under 18 under the Mental Health Act – these will need to include local agreements with the approved mental health practitioner/approved social worker and the local crisis intervention teams. (Where practical, the Mental Health Act assessment of young people under18 should include a Section 12 approved doctor with training in the assessment of adolescents (if possible a CAMHS consultant or specialist registrar)).

Powers of arrest and willingness to act

It is advisable that the local police agree with the emergency department the circumstances under which they will detain a member of the public who is behaving in an antisocial way in the emergency department. Until they are admitted, the emergency department is to be regarded as a public area. As such any law that applies to behaviour in a public place applies to the emergency department. This includes the use of Section 136. However, the police may have qualms about intervening in a medical setting, especially with a mentally ill person. This inhibition may be exaggerated in the case of a child or adolescent. It is thus important to have a policy agreed in writing and authorised by a senior officer.

Domestic violence

Each Local Authority should have a domestic violence policy agreed by the local domestic violence forum, and this should be available in the emergency department. This will require all staff who are aware of domestic violence to be proactive in supporting victims of domestic violence and protecting children who are exposed to witnessing or experiencing violence. If children are exposed or thought to be at significant risk of exposure, child protection procedures should be initiated. The domestic violence unit of the police (usually, in England at least, this is a subunit of the community police unit) are trained to deal sensitively with those involved in domestic violence, whether as victims or perpetrators.

Working with Social Services

There will be a duty social worker available at all times. Access and contact details need to be made clear to the emergency department, and to other first-line staff who may be part of the assessment of a child or adolescent.

Approved social workers

The Mental Health Act has no lower age limit. Under the Act's 2007 amendments, professionals other than social workers will be trained to make assessments alongside doctors for detention under the Act. They are now referred to as approved mental health practitioners. In all likelihood, most will continue to be approved social workers. Approved social workers are required to assess people of all ages and to know the law and how it applies to adolescents and children. However, it needs to be acknowledged that many approved social workers will have little experience of working with/interviewing young people and may have a reluctance to be involved in this kind of assessment without the support of their colleagues in the child and family team. Specialist dually trained child and family approved social workers are desirable, but are unfortunately in most parts of the UK a very rare commodity. There should be locally agreed policies for the assessment of children and adolescents under the Mental Health Act – in practice, these assessments may have to be conducted by both an approved social worker/approved mental health practitioner, and a child and family social worker, except out of hours when in practice an approved social worker working alone may have to suffice. In these cases, it is especially important for the approved social worker/approved mental health practitioner to have access to advice and consultation from a senior CAMHS professional. The local CAMHS should play a part in the training of approved mental health practitioners/approved social workers locally, and should at the very least check that there is a CAMHS module in the training.

Emergency placements

The social worker will have knowledge of and access to emergency placement of children and adolescents whose presentation to the emergency department is predicated on threats, dangers, inadequacies and/or stresses in their home placements or the absence of a reliable place to stay. Emergency placement through Social Services may obviate the need for a hospital admission in some cases. Frank and balanced discussion around the threshold for placement away from home for children and adolescents with challenging behaviour may have a sobering effect on them, and allow a more measured negotiation of compromises. Placements may include emergency foster placements, Social Services residential units, residential placements in the private or voluntary sector, or the negotiation of temporary safe placements with extended family of friends. There is a statutory duty on Social Services to provide for children under the age of 16 who have no (safe) home to live in – the predicament for 16- and 17-year-olds is well known, and it may be particularly important for there to be clear and explicit local agreements on the scope and threshold for Social Services' responsibility for this age group. The Children Act applies to anyone under the age of 18, and 16- and 17-year-olds may be defined as 'in need' under the Act (see also Chapter 7).

Child protection

The duty social worker must be involved in all cases of confirmed or suspected child abuse and neglect, if only to be consulted about the first steps to ensure the safety of the child, and to advise on the application of the local child protection policies and procedures. The emergency department will usually house or have access to the list of children subject to a child protection plan (child protection register) and this should be checked in all cases of children presenting to the emergency department. The social worker will also have access to the Social Services database, which may have useful information on children and families known to be at risk or requiring support services. The social worker's holistic assessment will also identify resilience and strengths in the family and in their support networks, which might be enhanced to reduce the risk of abuse or neglect. (See also Chapter 8, and Chapter 12, pp. 136–138.)

Family support

The duty social worker will be able to provide information on resources to support families in need. Knowing what resources may become available may reduce the sense of desperation of some families with ill or disturbing children, and allow them to cope a little longer and tolerate a little more in the short term. Resources may include: day centres; home-visiting support (social) workers; the potential for respite placements; women's refuge placements for families experiencing domestic violence and/or financial support; and support with getting appropriate social security benefits for families stressed by poverty and, specifically in the context of this document, where the stress of impoverishment is having an adverse effect on the mental health and socio-emotional development of the child. Asylum-seeking families unused to the social security system and especially where English is not their first language may need special assistance to navigate the regulations around subsistence funding and housing. Social Services will need to provide services for all 'unaccompanied minors'.

Services for children and adolescents with intellectual disabilities

In some areas, services for children and adolescents with intellectual disabilities is under the auspices of the Local Authority, and access to resources is controlled by Social Services. The duty social worker may have a useful and necessary role in the assessment of need of a child or adolescent with intellectual difficulties presenting to the emergency department with social or behavioural problems. Frustration or stress in the care environment of a non-verbal or verbally unskilled young person is likely to manifest as behavioural problems. Families and carers of children and adolescents with severe intellectual difficulties are often under enormous stress, especially where community support services are limited, and this should be borne in mind during the assessment so as not to make the parent/carer feel unduly blamed or inadequate.

Working with adult mental health services

The transition gap

Young people aged 16–18 years with mental health problems often fall within the gap between adult psychiatric services and CAMHS. Within the UK there is no consensus on how service boundaries should be delineated.

Eligibility for paediatric services is similarly inconsistent across and within jurisdictions. The NSF for children, young people and maternity services (Department of Health, 2004) and the Scottish framework (Scottish Executive, 2005) both propose that all children's services aim for a cut-off point of 18 years, but at present many CAMHS do not have the resources to achieve this, and there is debate within paediatrics about how best to implement this proposal.

Who assesses?

In the emergency department there is considerable variation throughout the UK as to who assesses the young person with mental health problems. Ideally, this should be a CAMHS professional, but especially out of hours, assessments of 16- and 17-year-olds may fall to the adult mental health duty team or paediatrician. Adult mental health first-line staff often have limited experience of child and adolescent mental health work, see young people too infrequently to develop the necessary experience and skills in working with this age group, and in some cases may not even have access to a CAMHS professional for telephone advice. Communication between CAMHS and adult mental health services is unfortunately often inadequate, even when the CAMHS and the adult mental health service are within the same trust, which is not inevitable. Although protocols for transition to adult services are now required under the NSF for mental health services (Department of Health, 1999), protocols for dealing with 16- and 17-year-olds seem to be the exception rather than the rule.

If admission is required

If a young person needs admission following assessment to a specialist psychiatric child and adolescent unit (often under a section of the Mental Health Act), a further structural problem becomes evident. There is a shortage of adolescent in-patient beds nationally. In some parts of the UK there are no beds for a considerable and impractical distance. Too few adolescent mental health in-patient beds are available and it is often very difficult to access these in an emergency situation. As a result, 16- and 17-year-olds requiring emergency admission are often admitted to an adult psychiatric ward. Again, adult psychiatric staff in these wards have little, if any, experience or training in child and adolescent mental health. These young people may be vulnerable to exploitation by adult patients and may well be very frightened in an adult setting as adult psychiatric wards are usually populated by adults with severe and often long-standing mental illnesses. Adult psychiatric wards have significant numbers of violent incidents, which again may frighten the young person and put them off future contact with mental health services.

The choice in these circumstances (where there are no available NHS specialist CAMHS beds) may be whether to admit the young patient to an adult ward, which at least is close to home and allows ongoing frequent and regular contact with family; to send them to (private) adolescent units at a considerable distance, disrupting their family and support networks; or to try to manage them in the community with the attendant risks, and often with overstretched community CAMHS providing inadequate services for such disturbed, disturbing and distressed young people and their families. It may be that, on balance, admission to an adult ward is the best and safest solution.

When admission is not required

Adult mental health first-line staff often do not know what facilities are available in CAMHS for a young person who has presented to the emergency department and indeed the appropriateness of these relative to the needs of the patient, for example waiting times for out-patient appointments. Child and adolescent, and adult mental health services in the community are set up in very different ways, catering for very different client groups. Few CAMHS have access to intensive facilities such as day hospitals or assertive outreach or home treatment teams.

Communication issues

It is widely agreed that communication between the services is very poor and that transition protocols may not exist. Local needs and priorities often determine how well established any links are. Some services have specialist workers who try to bridge the gap and in some cases joint working occurs. However, for the majority of services across the UK, communication is very poor and the young person may slip through the net.

Mental Health Act assessments

Further issues occur if an adolescent needs to be detained under the Mental Health Act, as few emergency staff (e.g. approved social workers and Section 12 approved doctors) have CAMHS experience or training.

Guidance and recommendations for practice

To address these issues, the Royal College of Psychiatrists have issued guidance for the management of general adult psychiatric junior doctors attending children and adolescents in the emergency department (Royal College of Psychiatrists, 2004a). This is encapsulated below.

Who to assess

Mental health staff attending the emergency department should be clear as to whom they are expected to see and what the expected outcome of the consultation will be. This should be agreed between clinical leads or heads of department locally and the agreement should be available to staff in the emergency department. There should be specific agreement about who will see a young person of 16 or 17 with an apparent mental health problem. There should also be a specific agreement about the circumstances under which a young person under 16 will be seen by an adult mental health professional (see also *Adult mental health first-line staff*, pp. 136–137 and *General adult/liaison consultant*, p. 143).

Who to consult

Mental health staff attending the emergency department should know whom they can call on for advice and guidance with respect to CAMHS patients they may need to see. Local arrangements for this are very variable, but the locally agreed form of specialist consultation (e.g. an on-call consultants' rota) and contact details should be in writing and available to staff in the emergency department.

Who to refer on to

Mental health staff attending the emergency department should know who else might usefully see the patient (and family) (and importantly, how to contact them) for further assessment, specific intervention or with a view to admission to a ward other than an adult mental health ward. (This would include, for example, paediatric services if they admit young people up to 18 years; the CAMHS senior trainee or consultant, who may be able to offer a crisis consultation and intervention; access an age-appropriate in-patient bed or suggest arrangements for urgent follow-up; or the duty or available social worker, who might arrange for social support or housing away from home.)

How to discharge a CAMHS patient

Discussion should take place with suitably qualified professionals (a CAMHS senior on-call professional if possible or a paediatric senior doctor if a CAMHS senior professional is not available according to local arrangements) before any decision regarding discharge from the emergency department takes place. Arrangements for follow-up should be in place at the point of discharge. The adult mental health worker should be aware of what local services are available for the young person, and if not, all the more reason to consult with a CAMHS professional or paediatric senior doctor. A 'catalogue' of local CAMHS should be available, giving a service description, waiting times (average) and contact details, and should be consulted if the discharge is to go ahead.

When admitting a young person under 18 to an adult ward

In circumstances where the only practicable solution is to admit a young person to an adult psychiatric in-patient unit, to make this as useful, safe and tolerable as possible, there should be a clearly agreed protocol between CAMHS and the adult mental health service for this exigency (as required by the 2007 amendments of the Mental Health Act (Department of Health 2008: Age-appropriate services, pp. 344–346)). This should specify that:

- the young person should be nursed separately in a cubicle, with one-to-one nursing by professionals who have CRB clearance to work with children;
- the family should be treated sensitively and sympathetically, be given full information about safeguards and be allowed extended visits if clinically appropriate;

- the ward should have a child protection policy and procedure for reporting, approved by the local child protection committee – there should be training of staff on this and the policy should be readily accessible;
- CAMHS should be alerted, if possible at the point of referral; CAMHS should provide consultation to the process of admission and assessment, and to clinical management from the outset, and offer an assessment, if possible, within the next working day;
- arrangements should be made at the earliest opportunity to transfer the patient to a more age-appropriate setting and where the balance of advantages determines that this is the better course of action.

Awareness of the effects of child abuse and child protection procedure

There is a considerable association between psychological distress in childhood and abuse of various types. Any suspicion of abuse needs to be taken seriously: in any case of suspected child abuse the local social work department must be contacted for advice. Contact numbers for the local Social Services child protection team should be available in all emergency departments. All staff should know when to and how to contact the local Social Services child protection team. All adult mental health workers require child protection training.

Children who are not the identified patient

In England and Wales, Section 11 of the Children Act 2004 makes it explicit that professionals attending adult patients with mental health problems have a responsibility to inform the local child protection team if they believe that there are children at risk of abuse or neglect. There is an understanding that confidentiality may have to be breached, but always seek advice before breaching confidentiality. The child protection team may be asked for their advice before or without revealing the patient's or family's identity. Scotland has identical duties of care. Furthermore, the Mental Health (Care and Treatment) (Scotland) Act 2003 places a duty of care on professionals to consider the needs of children in families where a parent/carer has a mental disorder. Children may sometimes accompany an injured or medically ill parent to the emergency department. They will have physical care needs as well as psychological support needs. These needs should not be medicalised: contact Social Services for help. Where well developed, the hospital chaplaincy can also be of considerable help. There should be a local agreement between the adult services the adult patient may present to (the emergency department and mental health services), children's services (CAMHS and paediatrics) and Social Services regarding cross-contact and procedures when an adult 'identified patient' brings a child with them to the emergency department. This needs to be subject to regular audit and review by all parties involved. This is best done through a standing inter-agency working group.

Self-harm in the under-16 age group

As well as possibly indicating suicidal intent, self-harm may also indicate a wide variety of other problems (including abuse) being experienced by the child. In contrast to the adult age group, current advice (National Institute for Health and Clinical Excellence, 2004) is that any child who self-harms should be admitted to hospital whether their physical state requires it or not. This would generally be to a paediatric ward. There should be a local protocol regarding self-harm in young people agreed between the various children's agencies. This should be available in the emergency department. This needs to be subject to regular audit and review by all parties involved. This is best done through a standing inter-agency working group.

Confirming age

When a young person attends the emergency department stating an age between 16 and 20, all efforts should be made to confirm their age. Unaccompanied minors (refugees) will sometimes have diminished their age to under 18 to get additional support and right to remain. If someone of 18 years or over is ultimately placed with minors, there will be child protection implications.

Adult mental health liaison

Adult mental health input to the emergency department should be undertaken by a relatively small multidisciplinary team of adult mental health staff, so that they can develop good working relationships with the emergency department staff, improve their experience and skills in dealing with the particular working environment in the emergency department, and develop expertise in dealing with particular groups (in this instance, young people).

Communication with CAMHS

There should be ongoing dialogue with the local CAMHS, with clear and unambiguous pathways of communication.

Communication with Social Services

There should also be an agreed point of contact with Social Services; ideally, Social Services staff should form part of the emergency department liaison team.

Interface with adult medical ward staff

Although this may change soon (as required by the NSF for children, young people and maternity services; Department of Health, 2004) it is still the practice in many areas for young people after they turn 16 to be accommodated on adult medical wards rather than paediatric wards. This may apply also to young people who have self-harmed, especially after an overdose, when they require ongoing medical intervention. Patients who self-harm may be at special risk on medical wards, where they have access to needles and medication left at other patients' bedsides. The safeguards recommended for adult psychiatric wards should also apply to medical wards.

Resources in the emergency department

Every emergency department should have interview facilities that are:

- safe – well-lit, not isolated, with availability of panic buttons and, if possible, with two exits, with furniture that cannot be thrown and no access to sharp objects;
- child- and adolescent-friendly (not medicalised);
- quiet and private, allowing for discussions that cannot be heard by those (e.g. parents) sitting outside;
- clean, uncluttered and reasonable comfortable;
- large enough to allow a meeting of professionals with the child/ adolescent and their family (space and seating for at least six people).

Department heads and managers should make themselves aware of the recommendations for ensuring a safe working environment (Royal College of Psychiatrists, 2004a: Safety, pp. 67–69).

Information management, medical records and databases

Rapid access to the child's or adolescent's medical records is essential for the provision of good and safe services. This may be complicated when more than one trust is involved as each has its own arrangements for storing medical records. Protocols need to be in place for access to notes in other trusts and notes kept on other sites (e.g. community clinics). Confidentiality is likely to be an inhibiting factor, and safeguarding confidentiality will be an important part of the protocol and procedure for accessing information from CAMHS sources. This will need the authorisation of the CAMHS consultant on call or a senior member of staff nominated by the CAMHS manager.

Electronic databases will in the future make it technically feasible for notes to be shared, but this ease of access will make it even more crucial for the portals of entry to be restricted in accordance with the Data Protection Act 1998 and the General Medical Council (2004) rules on confidentiality and disclosure of patient information.

Data should be collected in a way that allows audit studies to be facilitated.

Consideration should be given to a system for filing community care plans in accordance with the locally agreed community programme approach on young patients with mental health problems who are likely to attend the emergency department in crisis, including those classed as frequent attenders.

Some emergency departments operate a 'flag' or 'Green card' system, whereby identified highly vulnerable patients who are not likely to abuse the system are admitted more or less directly to the designated ward (usually this applies to paediatrics) with good results. This should be considered.

Access to the child protection register is a problem in some areas. All emergency departments should have direct access to their local register, but this is not always the case. In some areas, the register is held by the Local Authority and access to it is via the duty social worker, which can introduce an unacceptable delay in establishing whether the child is on the register or not. The hospital may serve more than one Local Authority area – the register may only be available for the area in which the hospital is situated (even when most of the patient population is drawn from the neighbouring area). There is currently no national child protection database and no system for electronically ascertaining whether the child is subject to child protection surveillance.

Commissioning of services

The commissioning primary care trusts in England, the local health boards in Wales, and in Scotland the health boards under the leadership of child health commissioners, should establish the following.

Arrangements for 24/7 emergency CAMHS cover to the emergency department

This should be a sustainable rota of senior CAMHS professionals in addition to psychiatric doctors and may include availability for direct intervention (usually provided by junior doctors or CAMHS liaison nurses) or, alternatively, availability for consultation on the telephone only (often this is provided by consultants or other suitably trained senior professionals) according to local resources.

Where this is provided by professionals other than consultant child and adolescent psychiatrists, appropriate supervision arrangements should be in place.

(See Department of Health, 2004: p.50; Department of Health, 2006: pp. 14–15.)

Services for 16- and 17-year-olds

Commissioners should ensure that agreements are in place between paediatric, adult mental health and CAMHS for the assessment and treatment of 16- and 17-year-olds, including agreeing thresholds for admission and the provision of suitable designated beds if they need admission.

If they are to be admitted to an adult mental health bed, written arrangements for this to happen in a way that best protects the young person from abuse and humiliation should be in place. This should include advice on dealing with the young person's and the family's understandable fears and misgivings. The preferred arrangement would be for the young person to be nursed in a single room with one-to-one nursing by nurses who have been CRB checked, and who have access to advice from a CAMHS nurse (preferably) or another suitable CAMHS professional. The young person should be transferred to a designated adolescent unit bed at the earliest opportunity. (See also Department of Health, 2004.)

Emergency psychiatric in-patient provision

Commissioners should ensure that local and regional arrangements for the emergency admission of a child or adolescent are in place and known to the emergency department. Children under 16 needing admission should, whenever possible, be admitted to a paediatric ward. Protocols including inclusion and exclusion criteria for this should be written and available to on-call paediatric junior staff seeing the child in the emergency department. What have become standard and recommended arrangements for all children under 16 who self-harm to be admitted to paediatrics may need to be reviewed with the shift in paediatric provision to more ambulatory care and fewer in-patient beds.

With the harmonisation of all children's services to include all those under 18 years, according to the NSF for children, young people and maternity services (Department of Health, 2004), commissioners should encourage the development of adolescent-specific medical (paediatric) services and in-patient resources. These should include the capacity to admit young people with mental health problems, including self-harm, as long as the risks of admitting them do not impede the medical treatment of other patients (i.e. they should not be in a highly disturbed state or dangerous).

Commissioners are now required by law to block-purchase specialist acute adolescent unit beds or make available sufficient funds for acquiring beds in the private sector in an emergency. The number of beds should be established by a needs assessment, taking into account the fluctuations in bed utilisation over at least 3 years. The Royal College of Psychiatry's Child and Adolescent Faculty have recently published a needs-based guide for commissioners on likely bed numbers for this purpose (Royal College of Psychiatrists, 2006b: pp. 12–13). Each strategic health sector should move to commission, through a consortium of primary care trusts, its own NHS acute adolescent in-patient facility. In Scotland, health boards and regional planning groups would commission these services.

Waiting times

In practice, the 4 h waiting time (more appositely, the completed intervention time) in the emergency department for resolution of a mental health crisis for children and adolescents is in many cases impractical, and may lead to ineffective, minimising or unduly restrictive outcomes. Exclusion criteria will need to be agreed with commissioners and if necessary with the strategic health authorities who are charged with performance monitoring. It may be advisable to have locally agreed response times for each of triage, for first assessment by paediatric first-line staff (for under 16s and, where applicable, all under 18s), for mental health first-line staff (where there is agreement to see over 16s) and for CAMHS consultation.

Interpreting services

Adequate interpreting services should be available as and when required (see Chapter 9).

References

Academy of Medical Royal Colleges (2008) *Managing Urgent Mental Health Needs in the Acute Trust: A Guide by Practitioners for Managers and Commissioners in England and Wales*. Academy of Medical Royal Colleges.

Allen, M. H. (1996) Definitive treatment in the psychiatric emergency service. *Psychiatric Quarterly*, **67**, 247–262.

Behar, L. J. & Shrier, D. K. (1995) Child and adolescent psychiatric emergencies: referral and discharge patterns. *New Jersey Medicine*, **92**, 236–239.

Department for Constitutional Affairs (2007) *Mental Capacity Act 2005 Code of Practice*. TSO (The Stationery Office).

Department of Health (1999) *National Service Framework for Mental Health: Modern Standards and Service Models*. TSO (The Stationery Office) (http://www.dh.gov.uk/en/Publicationsandstatistics/Publications/PublicationsPolicyAndGuidance/DH_4009598).

Department of Health (2003a) *Confidentiality: NHS Code of Practice*. TSO (The Stationery Office) (http://www.dh.gov.uk/en/Publicationsandstatistics/Publications/PublicationsPolicyAndGuidance/DH_4069253).

Department of Health (2003b) *What To Do If You're Worried A Child Is Being Abused*. HM Government (http://www.dh.gov.uk/en/Publicationsandstatistics/Lettersandcirculars/LocalAuthorityCirculars/AllLocalAuthority/DH_4003423).

Department of Health (2004) *National Service Framework for Children, Young People and Maternity Services. Executive Summary*. TSO (The Stationery Office) (http://www.dh.gov.uk/en/Publicationsandstatistics/Publications/PublicationsPolicyandGuidance/DH_4089100).

Department of Health (2006) *Report on the Implementation of Standard 9 of the National Service Framework for Children, Young People and Maternity Services*. TSO (The Stationery Office) (http://www.dh.gov.uk/en/Publicationsandstatistics/Publications/PublicationsPolicyAndGuidance/DH_062778).

Department of Health (2008) *Code of Practice. Mental Health Act 1983*. TSO (The Stationary Office).

Fox, C. & Hawton, K. (2004) *Deliberate Self-Harm in Adolescence*. Jessica Kingsley.

General Medical Council (2004) *Confidentiality: protecting and providing information*. GMC (http://www.gmc-uk.org/guidance/current/library/confidentiality.asp).

Greenfield, B., Hechtman, L. & Tremblay, C. (1995) Short-term efficacy of internventions by a youth crisis team. *Canadian Journal of Psychiatry*, **40**, 320–324.

Gutterman, E. M., Markowitz, J. S., LoConte, J. S., *et al* (1993) Determinants for hospitalisation from an emergency mental health service. *Journal of the American Academy of Child and Adolescent Psychiatry*, **32**, 114–122.

Hawton, K., Rodham, K., Evans, E., *et al* (2002) Deliberate self-harm in adolescents: self-report survey in schools in England. *BMJ*, **325**, 1207–1211.

Healthcare Commission (2006) *Improvement Review: Services for Children in Hospital.* Healthcare Commission (http://www.healthcarecommission.org.uk/_db/_documents/ Improvement_review_of_services_for_children_in_hospital.pdf).

Healy, E., Saha, S., Subotsky, F., *et al* (2002) Emergency presentations to an inner-city adolescent psychiatric service. *Journal of Adolescence,* **25**, 397–404.

HM Government (2006) *Working Together to Safeguard Children.* TSO (The Stationery Office) (http://www.everychildmatters.gov.uk/resources-and-practice/IG00060/).

Kingsbury, S. (1996) PATHOS: a screening instrument for adolescent overdose: a research note. *Journal of Child Psychology and Psychiatry,* **37**, 609–611.

Malek, M. & Joughin, C. (eds) (2004) *Child and Adolescent Mental Health Services for Children and Adolescents from Minority Ethnic Groups.* College Research Unit/Focus Project, Royal College of Psychiatrists.

Mental Health Foundation (2006) *Truth Hurts. Report of the National Inquiry into Self-harm Among Young People.* Mental Health Foundation (http://www.mentalhealth.org.uk/ publications/?EntryId5=38712).

National Institute for Health and Clinical Excellence (2004) *Self-Harm: The Short-Term Physical and Psychological Management and Secondary Prevention of Self-Harm in Primary and Secondary Care.* NICE (http://www.nice.org.uk/nicemedia/pdf/CG016NICEguideline. pdf).

National Institute for Mental Health in England (2006) *The Social Work Contribution to Mental Health Services: The Future Direction.* NIMHE.

Office for National Statistics (2005) *Mental Health of Children and Young People in Great Britain, 2004.* TSO (The Stationery Office).

Parker, C. & Rose, G. (2004) *Guidelines for Rapid Control of Acuyely Disturbed Younger Patients (Aged 6–17 Years).* United Kingdom Psychiatric Pharmacy Group (http://www.ukppg. org.uk/04-ape-younger-cnwl.pdf).

Pumariega, A. J. & Winters, N. C. (2003) Trends and shifting ecologies. Part II. *Child and Adolescent Psychiatric Clinics of North America,* **12**, 779–793.

Pierce, D. W. (1977) Suicidal intent in self-injury. *British Journal of Psychiatry,* **130**, 377–385.

Re W (A Minor) (Wardship: Medical Treatment) [1992] 4 AllER 627, CA.

Reilly, P. L., Simpson, D. A., Sprod, R., *et al* (1988) Assessing the conscious level in infants and young children: a paediatric version of the Glasgow Coma Scale. *Child's Nervous System,* **4**, 30–33.

Royal College of Paediatrics and Child Health (2004) *Responsibilities of doctors in child protection cases with regard to confidentiality.* Royal College of Paediatrics and Child Health.

Royal College Paediatrics and Child Health (2006) *Child Protection Companion.* Royal College of Paediatrics and Child Health.

Royal College of Psychiatrists (1998) *Managing Deliberate Self-Harm in Young People. Council Report CR64.* Royal College of Psychiatrists (http://www.rcpsych.ac.uk/files/pdfversion/ cr64.pdf).

Royal College of Psychiatrists (2004a) *Psychiatric Services to Accident and Emergency Departments. Council Report CR118.* Royal College of Psychiatrists (http://www.rcpsych. ac.uk/files/pdfversion/cr118.pdf).

Royal College of Psychiatrists (2004b) *Assessment Following Self-harm in Adults. Council Report CR122.* Royal College of Psychiatrists (http://www.rcpsych.ac.uk/files/pdfversion/ cr122.pdf).

Royal College of Psychiatrists (2006a) *Child and Adolescent Mental Health Problems in the Emergency Department and the Services to Deal with These.* Royal College of Psychiatrists (http://www.rcpsych.ac.uk/college/faculties/childandadolescent/newsandinformation. aspx).

Royal College of Psychiatrists (2006b) *Building and Sustaining Specialist Child and Adolescent Mental Health Services. Council Report CR137.* Royal College of Psychiatrists (http://www. rcpsych.ac.uk/files/pdfversion/CR137.pdf).

Scottish Executive (2005) *The Mental Health of Children and Young People: A Framework for Promotion, Prevention and Care*. Scottish Executive.

Skegg, K. (2005) Self-harm. *Lancet*, **366**, 1471–1483.

Spender, Q. (2007) Assessment of adolescent self-harm. *Paediatrics and Child Health*, **17**, 448–453.

Storey, P. & Statham, J. (2007) *Meeting the Target: Providing on-call and 24-hour Specialist Cover in Child and Adolescent Mental Health Services*. Thomas Coram Research Unit, Institute of Education.

Teasdale, G. & Jennett, B. (1974) Assessment of coma and impaired consciousness. A practical scale. *Lancet*, **2**, 81–84.

Thomas, L. E. (2003) Trends and shifting ecologies. Part I. *Child and Adolescent Psychiatric Clinics of North America*, **12**, 599–611.

Appendix I
Recommendations of the Joint Colleges Working Group[1] on CAMHS in the emergency department[2]

Tony Kaplan

General

- Services to meet the needs of children and adolescents under the age of 18 with mental health emergencies and their families should be expanded and improved in line with increased demand.
- Evidence-based research should be funded urgently into effective crisis interventions and models of service delivery for this target group. Clinical descriptive and theoretical papers should be encouraged by journal editors at this preliminary stage to address the paucity of literature in this vital area of practice and to try to identify good practice principles.
- The findings of the Department of Health funded study by the Thomas Coram Foundation (Storey & Statham, 2007) into current delivery of 24/7 CAMHS should be widely distributed.
- Best practice should be aspired to by clinicians, provider managers and commissioners, with the recognition that realistically local provision will always be a compromise taking into account the pragmatics of current resources and the developmental trajectory of the service organisations involved. Beacons of good practice should be championed by national mental health (and children's health) organisations such as Young Minds, the National Institute for Mental Health in England, the Scottish Intercollegiate Guidelines Network (SIGN), and the Mental Health Foundation, as well as by the Department of Health in England, through, for example, the NSF implementation group for England to help drive development forward.

---

1. Royal College of Psychiatrists, Royal College of Paediatrics & Child Health, and College of Emergency Medicine.
2. Royal College of Psychiatrists (2006a) *Child and Adolescent Mental Health Problems in the Emergency Department, and the Services to Deal with These*. Royal College of Psychiatrists.

- Services should be child and adolescent-friendly and responsive to the needs and feelings of families.
- Services should be provided in a culturally sensitive way.
- The development of hospital-based services should be underpinned by the development of good community crisis intervention and home treatment services in line with the NICE and SIGN guidelines on early intervention for mental health problems.
- Paediatric, CAMHS and Social Services should be harmonised at the earliest possible time with regard to age eligibility up to 18 years, in line with the NSF for children, young people and maternity services (Department of Health, 2004), and the *Framework for Promotion, Prevention and Care* (Scottish Executive, 2005) in Scotland. Accordingly, there should be greater availability of adolescent-specific in-patient services and wards within paediatrics and child health.

Competencies

- All professionals who intervene in the crisis of urgent mental health problems for children, adolescents and their families should have the competencies detailed in the relevant section of this document (see Chapter 12) for each branch of service, know the limits of their competence, know who to call on for advice when this threshold is reached, know who to refer on to, and know how to refer on efficiently to the professional or branches of service best placed to attend to the difficulties presented by child and family so as to relieve distress most effectively.
- The Postgraduate Medical Education and Training Board (PMETB) together with the the Royal College of Psychiatrists, the Royal College of Paediatrics and Child Health, and the College of Emergency Medicine should all ensure that affiliated (junior) doctors assessing children and adolescents in the emergency setting receive adequate training in order to have sufficient knowledge of the presentation of mental health problems in this age group to make an initial (working) diagnostic formulation, risk assessment and risk management plan.
- All professionals required to make decisions about the care and treatment of children and adolescents should have a working understanding of the issues of consent and 'mental capacity' (competence) and the legal framework for children and adolescents, especially with regard to parental responsibility and the child's right to confidentiality.
- Child and adolescent psychiatrists should, in addition, have specialist knowledge regarding the use of psychotropic medication, especially with reference to rapid tranquillisation in children and adolescents.
- Child and adolescent psychiatrists should have specialist knowledge and recognised training in the applications of the Mental Health Act or equivalent legislation within their jurisdiction.

163

- The duty social worker or at least the social worker in the emergency department should, in cases of family or social breakdown, have the skills to intervene to prevent hospitalisation where safe and appropriate, if possible returning the child or adolescent home or to a kinship-based placement, and detailed local knowledge about emergency social placements, where this is not possible.

Training

- The Child and Adolescent Faculty of the Royal College of Psychiatrists through its Education and Training Committee, and in partnership with PMETB, should ensure that the theoretical frameworks, methodologies and practices of crisis intervention with children and adolescents and their families is a core module on the curriculum of training for child psychiatry trainees.
- It is the duty of the managers within each branch of service to ensure that training on child protection is mandatory and kept up to date for all staff.
- Managers should ensure that training on diversity, cultural awareness and sensitivity, and anti-discriminatory practice is regularly made available to all first-line staff.

Organisation and working arrangements

- Emergency services and departments should have in place robust working arrangements to ensure effective and efficient inter-agency, inter-departmental and interdisciplinary coordination and communication. These should be signed up to by primary care referrers to the services, the police and ambulance services, voluntary sector services where relevant, the emergency department, adult mental health services, paediatrics and CAMHS liaison, and community and Tier 4 services. This is particularly important in those health boards where, as a result of a lack of investment, local specialist CAMHS are unable to provide a service up to a young person's 18th birthday.
- Working arrangements should include written agreements and joint protocols (for interventions and cross-referral), and an agreed competency framework, as outlined in this document.
- Management arrangements should including the establishment of an emergency services/department liaison committee, with clearly agreed roles and responsibilities of senior professionals, including responsibility for training and induction of junior staff, and of new, agency or locum staff.
- Where there is a separate paediatric emergency service/department, a discreet paediatric liaison committee structure, chaired jointly by a paediatric and a CAMHS consultant, is recommended, as long as the

needs of young people of 16 and 17 are included, especially where paediatric services do not yet serve young people over 16.

- There should be clear written agreements in place for admission to in-patient CAMHS, including referral procedure, thresholds for admission, inclusion and exclusion criteria, information available to young people and their carers, arrangements for transfer and emergency funding authorisation.

- Emergency departments must have ready access to a duty social worker at all times, for advice regarding statutory interventions and matters of children's and mental health law, and consultation and interventions where necessary with regard to child protection and the emergency placement of children and adolescents away from home in a non-medical setting.

- Emergency department, paediatric and CAMHS staff and social workers working in the emergency department must have access to the child protection register or its equivalent.

- The locally agreed child protection policy and procedure should be easily available for reference to all staff dealing with children and adolescents in the emergency department. Consultation, supervision and training on child protection procedures must be available in each service.

- There should be an agreed and functioning domestic violence policy in the emergency department, and in so far as this effects children, domestic violence should elicit a child protection response from the professionals dealing with such cases, even when the child has not been injured.

- The director of Social Services should take responsibility for ensuring that Social Services has within its stock of residential resources suitable accommodation for young people of 16 and 17 with emotional and behavioural problems of a kind that do not warrant specialist in-patient psychiatric care.

- Whether the emergency department is suitable as a designated place of safety for adolescents who may be violent needs to be agreed locally between the emergency department, paediatrics, CAMHS, adult mental health services, Social Services and the police, and confirmed in writing. It is vital that if the paediatric emergency department is to be used in this way, the police agree to wait to provide assistance. Within this agreement there should be provision for the emergency assessment of disturbed teenagers in police custody if they are so violent they cannot safely be brought to the hospital. The police's powers of arrest and willingness to act in this setting, even with young people who appear to be unwell, must be agreed in writing and authorised by a senior officer.

- The recommendations for ensuring a safe working environment contained in the College Report CR118 are endorsed (Royal College of Psychiatrists, 2004a: Safety, pp. 67–69).

- Emergency department managers must have the systems in place to allow rapid access to the child's or adolescent's medical records, which should include mechanisms and protocols for access to notes in other trusts, and notes kept on other sites (e.g. community clinics), and which respect the child and family's right to confidentiality.
- There should be in each emergency department an agreed system for filing in an accessible way any existing community care plans, in accordance with the care programme approach, on young patients who are likely to attend the emergency department in crisis.
- Data on all cases seen in the emergency department should be collected in a way that allows for audit by the liaison committee.

Resources

- Emergency departments and paediatric emergency departments should provide interview facilities for the assessment of children and adolescents presenting with mental health crises that are safe, child- and adolescent-friendly, quiet and private, clean and reasonably comfortable, and large enough to allow a meeting of professionals with the child/adolescent and their family.
- Commissioners should provide adequate funding for, or at least ensure that emergency departments provide adequately for, professionally accredited interpreting and translation services for children, adolescents and families who are not fluent in English, accessible in an emergency. Especially in a crisis, the bias when in doubt should be to use an interpreter, and where available, the 'link worker' for that local community, and this should not be limited by cost.

Commissioning

- Health commissioners should ensure that their local emergency departments have in place the availability of urgent CAMHS telephone consultation within a reasonable time around the clock by senior CAMHS professionals on a sustainable rota (and agreement within this about where clinical responsibility rests), and arrangements in place for a specialist CAMHS assessment and intervention for children, adolescents and their carers within the next working day, and that where necessary, additional funding is made available for this.
- Health commissioners should ensure that there are sufficient specialist (Tier 4 CAMHS) in-patient beds for children and adolescents in crisis who need admission and who cannot be managed or treated effectively on a paediatric ward. In-patient treatment where necessary should be as close to the patient's home as possible, unless safety or super-specialist considerations override this and the decision is made in collaboration with the patient and those with parental responsibility.

- Commissioners should ensure that there are services to meet the needs of 16- and 17-year-olds in crisis. In Scotland, commissioners should provide sufficient resources to specialist CAMHS to allow adherence with the recommendations of the Mental Health (Care and Treatment) (Scotland) Act 2003.
- Hospital managers and commissioners should agree in advance that the maximum 4 h waiting time in the emergency department should be exceeded without penalty in the patient's interest where this will allow the time necessary for arrangements to be made for transfer to tertiary units, including specialist adolescent units or Social Services placements, where these are more appropriate.

Practice

- All children and adolescents presenting with unusual mental states and behaviour should have a physical examination by a paediatrician, and if indicated, special investigations, to rule out organic underlying causes.
- Young people who self-harm should be triaged rapidly by emergency department staff trained to deal with this problem in this age group, and every effort should be made to ensure that they are supported to stay in the emergency department for attention to their emotional state beyond attention to their physical (medical/surgical) problems. All young people under 16 presenting at the emergency department having self-harmed should be admitted to the paediatric ward under a consultant paediatrician to be assessed as soon as possible or at least within the next working day by a suitably qualified professional, trained to assess teenagers at risk of suicide and to intervene to reduce risk and to make a robust risk management plan. Where local arrangements allow, all 16- and 17-year-olds who self-harm should also be admitted, unless they have been assessed by the duty (adult) or CAMHS psychiatrist and found to be at low risk of suicide, and arrangements can be reliably made to prevent escalation of risk, if discharged, to be followed up in the community.
- No young person under 18 should be admitted to an adult mental health service bed when an adolescent unit bed is available within a reasonable distance, unless there is very good reason to do so, or unless this is the freely expressed preference of the older adolescent.
- Where young people are admitted to an adult mental health service bed for reasons of practicality or safety, this must be seen as a temporary solution only, and there should always be locally agreed protocols for this exigency, including written agreements for the young person to be accommodated separately with continuous one-to-one nursing care by staff who have been CRB checked as having no offences against children, and with the active daily involvement of a CAMHS consultant.

- The Royal College of Psychiatrists guidance for general psychiatrists and junior doctors attending children and adolescents in the emergency department is endorsed (Royal College of Psychiatrists, 2006a).
- Locally agreed protocols for transition from CAMHS to adult mental health services should be in place and available also to emergency department staff referring on.
- All cases involving actual or suspected abuse or neglect of a child should be referred to the duty or child protection social worker.
- There should be protocols for the emergency assessment of young people under the Mental Health Act or equivalent legislation. Where possible, this should include a specialist social worker, dually trained and accredited to work with children and families and to apply mental health legal restrictions, and an approved child and adolescent consultant or specialist registrar. A CAMHS consultant should be nominated in each trust to take the lead in adolescent psychiatry, and should ensure that the local training and updating of approved social workers or their equivalent includes a CAMHS module, and should provide this with other members of the CAMHS multidisciplinary team if necessary.
- The emergency department management team (or the paediatric management team in the case of a paediatric emergency department) should ensure that there is an agreed policy on dealing with violent incidents, including an agreed policy on restraining children and adolescents and regular accredited training for all staff who may be required to restrain safely a child or adolescent. Such child-centred training must include non-physical management of violence or potential violence, so-called de-escalation, and this should always be used in preference to physical restraint, where this is safe. Rapid tranquillisation should only be used as a last resort, and should be done in consultation with a CAMHS consultant or other delegated psychiatrists with or in higher training in child and adolescent psychiatry, and in accordance with the protocol contained in this document. The general recommendations in the College Report CR118 (Royal College of Psychiatrists, 2004a: pp. 44–46) on preventing and dealing with violence in the emergency department in people with mental health problems are supported to the extent that they apply to young people and their families.
- Systems should be in place to recognise frequent attenders, their particular patterns of presentation, risks involved and interventions that may ameliorate their distress, and attend helpfully to their help-seeking behaviour. The recommendations in the College Report CR118 (Royal College of Psychiatrists, 2004a; pp. 48–49) are endorsed.

Appendix II
Mental state examination checklist

Tony Kaplan

Behaviour

- Presentation/appearance
- Activity/arousal
- Posture/breathing/eye contact
- Appropriateness/congruence
- Mannerisms
- Tics/restlessness
- Distractibility/attention
- Inhibition/withdrawal
- Disinhibition

Relatedness

- 'Engageability'/rapport
- Friendliness/hostility
- Suspiciousness/wariness
- Humour
- Responsiveness

Speech

- Speed
- Flow
- Cadence/inflection
- Hesitancy/redundancy/passivity
- Fullness/richness
- Coherence
- Speech mannerisms/jargon/stiltedness
- Speech sounds/vocal tics
- Rhyming/slang associations
- Loose associations
- Flight of ideas/ derailments (formal thought disorder)
- Neologisms
- Scatology/excessive swearing

Affect

- Evident mood
    - relaxed/calm
    - tense/anxious
    - irritable
    - sad/depressed
    - elated
    - suspicious
    - perplexed
    - flattened/blunted affect
    - emotional constriction
    - limited range/responsiveness
    - dissociated/trance-like state
- Recent mood
    - anxiety/panic
    - depression/sadness
    - elation
    - paranoid
    - stamina
- History of self-harm/suicidality
- Biological symptoms of depression
- Sleep
    - initial insomnia
    - disrupted sleep
    - early morning waking
    - somnolence
    - nightmares/night terrors
    - sleep walking/talking
    - nocturnal enuresis
- Appetite
    - food: loss of appetite/loss of weight; inhibited appetite/restriction; eating attitudes/body image
    - enjoyable activity
    - (sex)
- Somatic symptoms of anxiety – panic
- Psychosomatic symptoms

Thought pattern/thinking

- Preoccupation/worry
- Obsessional rumination
    - compulsive behaviour/rituals
- Fears and phobias
- Depressive thinking
    - hopelessness
    - helplessness
    - pessimism/ negative selectivity
    - self-blame/self-criticism
    - suicidality
    - depressive anger/self-harm

- Thought disorder
  - formal thought disorder, including incoherence, derailments/knight's move thinking, loosening of associations/slang associations
  - thought alienation
  - thought broadcast/ transfer/mind-reading
  - thought blocking/stopping
- Coping thoughts/strategies

Ideation

- Catastrophic ideation
- Ideas of reference
- Intrusive memories/images
- Delusions
  - depressive delusions
  - paranoid delusions
  - grandiose delusions

Perception

- Hallucinations
  - auditory
  - visual
  - olfactory
  - kinaesthetic
  - gustatory
- Pseudohallucinations
- Dissociation
  - depersonalisation
  - derealisation
  - anaesthesia (numbing) – physical, affective

Cognitive functioning

- Orientation
- Concentration
- Memory
- Level of consciousness

Insight

Motivation to change

Appendix III
Mental Health Act 2007:
brief guide

Section	Comment
Section 136	*Removal by police from a public place to a place of safety.* *Duration of detention: 72h.*
Procedure	If it appears to a police officer that a person in a public place is 'suffering from a mental disorder' and is 'in immediate need of care or control', he can take that person to a 'place of safety'. The person should be examined by a doctor and interviewed by an approved mental health practitioner (previously an approved social worker).
Section 5	*Compulsory detention of informal patients already admitted to hospital.* *Duration of detention: by doctor, 72h (Section 5.2); by nurse, 6h (Section 5.4).* *Not applicable unless patient already admitted to a bed.*
Procedure	The duty doctor as nominated deputy of the responsible medical officer/responsible clinician must inform the hospital managers that the patient is suffering from a mental disorder to such a degree that it is necessary for his health or safety or for the protection of others for him to be immediately restrained from leaving the hospital. **Note**: The holding power only starts after the Section has been received by the hospital managers.
Section 4	*Admission for assessment in cases of emergency.* *Duration: 72h.*
Procedure	One doctor must confirm: • an urgent necessity that the patient should be admitted and detained for assessment; and • waiting for a second doctor to confirm the need for admission would involve undesirable delay.
Application	By the nearest relative or the approved mental health practitioner (previously an approved social worker). The applicant must have seen the patient within the last 24h. **Note**: the recommendation should clarify the circumstances of the emergency. The doctor must have seen the patient within 24h prior to admission.
Discharge	• Responsible medical officer/responsible clinician • Three members of the hospital management • The nearest relative (must give 72h notice) • Mental health review tribunal • After expiry of the period of detention while absent without leave (Section 18) **Note**: A responsible medical officer/responsible clinician can prevent the nearest relative from discharging the patient by making a report to the hospital managers.
Section 2	*Admission to hospital for assessment followed by treatment.* *Duration of detention: 28 days.*
Procedure	Two doctors must confirm in writing that: • the patient has a mental disorder of a nature or degree that warrants detention in hospital for assessment (or assessment followed by treatment); and

Section	Comment
	• the patient ought to be so detained in the interests of his own health or safety or with the view to the protection of others.
Application	By the nearest relative or the approved mental health practitioner (previously an approved social worker). Applicant must have seen the patient within 14 days prior to the date of application.
	Note: One of the practitioners should be approved as having 'special experience in the diagnosis or treatment of mental disorder'. When the two practitioners examine the patient separately, not more than 5 days must have elapsed between the two examinations and the last one must have taken place in the 14 days prior to the application. One of the practitioners should, if practicable, have had previous acquaintance with the patient.
Discharge	As per Section 4.
Section 3	*Admission to hospital for treatment.* *Duration: up to 6 months.*
Procedure	Two doctors must confirm in writing that: • the patient is suffering from a mental disorder (being 'any disorder of mind or brain'); and • his mental disorder is of a nature or degree that makes it appropriate for him to receive treatment in hospital; and • that appropriate treatment is available in the hospital to which he will be detained.
	Note: Both medical certificates must contain one form of disorder in common. In the case of psychopathic disorder or mental impairment, such treatment has the purpose of alleviating or preventing a worsening of the disorder or one of its manifestations. It is necessary for the health or safety of the patient or for the protection of other persons that he should receive such treatment, and it cannot be provided unless he is detained under this Section.
Application	As per Section 2.
Discharge	• Responsible medical officer/responsible clinician • Three members of the hospital management • The nearest relative (must give 72 h notice) • Mental health review tribunal • Aafter 28 days absent without leave • After 6 months continuously absent with leave
	Note: A responsible medical officer/responsible clinician can bar discharge by the nearest relative. The relative then has 28 days to apply to a mental health review tribunal.

Appendix IV
Ten essential shared competencies for mental health practice[1]

1   **Working in partnership**
    Developing and maintaining constructive working relationships with service users, carers, families, colleagues, lay people and wider community networks. Working positively with any tensions created by conflicts of interest or aspiration that may arise between the partners in care.

2   **Respecting diversity**
    Working in partnership with service users, carers, families and colleagues to provide care and interventions that not only make a positive difference but also do so in ways that respect and value diversity including age, race, culture, disability, gender, spirituality and sexuality.

3   **Practising ethically**
    Recognising the rights and aspirations of service users and their families, acknowledging power differentials and minimising them whenever possible. Providing treatment and care that is accountable to service users and carers within the boundaries prescribed by national (professional), legal and local codes of ethical practice.

4   **Challenging inequality**
    Addressing the causes and consequences of stigma, discrimination, social inequality and exclusion on service users, carers and mental health services. Creating, developing or maintaining valued social roles for people in the communities they come from.

5   **Promoting recovery**
    Working in partnership to provide care and treatment that enables service users and carers to tackle mental health problems with hope and optimism and to work towards a valued lifestyle within and beyond the limits of any mental health problem.

---

1. National Institute for Mental Health in England (2006*a*) *The Ten Essential Shared Capabilities: A Framework for the Whole of the Mental Health Workforce.* NIMHE.

6   **Identifying people's needs and strengths**
     Working in partnership to gather information to agree health and social
     care needs in the context of the preferred lifestyle and aspirations of
     service users their families, carers and friends.

7   **Providing service user centred care**
     Negotiating achievable and meaningful goals; primarily from the
     perspective of service users and their families. Influencing and seeking
     the means to achieve these goals and clarifying the responsibilities
     of the people who will provide any help that is needed, including
     systematically evaluating outcomes and achievements.

8   **Making a difference**
     Facilitating access to and delivering the best quality, evidence-based,
     values-based health and social care interventions to meet the needs
     and aspirations of service users and their families and carers.

9   **Promoting safety and positive risk taking**
     Empowering the person to decide the level of risk they are prepared
     to take with their health and safety. This includes working with the
     tension between promoting safety and positive risk taking, including
     assessing and dealing with possible risks for service users, carers,
     family members, and the wider public.

10   **Personal development and learning**
     Keeping up to date with changes in practice and participating in
     lifelong learning, personal and professional development for oneself
     and colleagues through supervision, appraisal and reflective practice.

Appendix V
Protocols[1]

Example 1: Southampton University Teaching Hospital

Attempted suicide/overdose (Fig. V.i)

Admission

- When presented with any form of attempted suicide/overdose, it is important to ask about suicidal ideas and intent.
- Anyone under 18 years who expresses any suicidal intent or ideas must be admitted.
- Anyone under 16 years who has attempted to overdose must be admitted, irrespective of how dangerous the attempt was.
- Anyone who refuses admission should be discussed with the on-call child and adolescent psychiatrist:
  - via switchboard if out of hours/weekends
  - via paediatric liaison team (Monday to Friday)
  - it is appropriate to use security to stop someone discharging themselves before being assessed using the common law/Children Act, if the level of concern warrants it.

Any young person up to the age of 18 years, even if on the adult ward, will be cared for jointly by the CAMHS team. The medical consultant responsible for the young person will be dependent on whether the young person is admitted to an adult or paediatric ward.

If not admitted

Up to 16th birthday
- Inform GP.
- If known to local psychiatry/social worker teams it would be helpful for them to be informed the next working day (consider referral if not known).

---

1. Southampton University Teaching Hospital protocol submitted by Josie Brown. Whittington Hospital protocol submitted by Sebastian Kraemer.

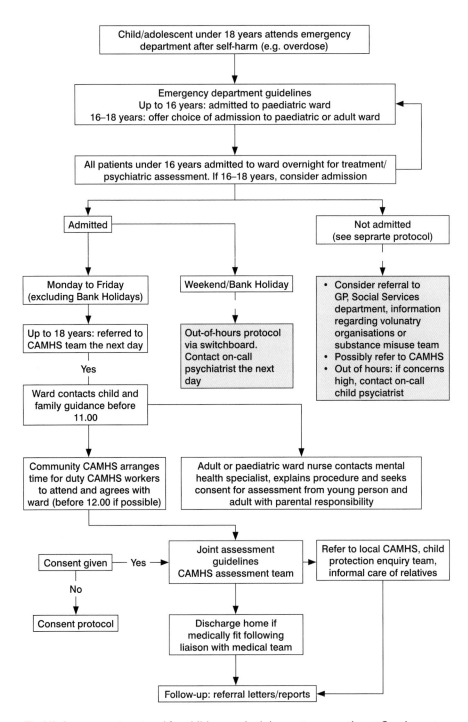

Fig. V.i Assessment protocol for children and adolescents presenting at Southampton University Teaching Hospital following self-harm. CAMHS, child and adolescent mental health services; GP, general practitioner.

- Inform young person of voluntary services (Box V.i).
- Ensure discharge is to a safe environment and responsible adult.
- Ensure parents are informed.

Between 16th and 18th birthday

- Inform GP.
- If known to local psychiatry/social worker teams it would be helpful for them to be informed the next working day (consider referral if not known).
- Inform young person of voluntary services (Box V.i).
- If you feel the young person is at continuing risk consider informing the parents, even if against the young persons wishes.
- If unsure, discuss with the psychiatry team.

Alcohol intoxication

If the young person scores ≤14 on the Glasgow Coma Scale, they need to be admitted (emergency department guidelines).

Most young people that present with alcohol intoxication do so because they are feeling unwell. Some may have underlying individual or family problems that need attention.

If, during the assessment, psychological concerns are raised, then consider admission.

- The younger the child, the greater your concern should be.
- If you believe the young person is in immediate danger (from themselves or others) consider admission.

Box V.i Useful services/organisations to contact

- Paediatric liaison team (Monday to Friday)
- On-call child and adolescent psychiatrist (out of hours/weekend/Bank Holiday via hospital switchboard)
- Brookvale Adolescent Service
- Young People's Substance Misuse Service
- Break Out Lesbian and Gay Youth Project
- Eating disorders helpline
- Solent lesbian and gay helpline
- Emergency contraception helpline
- The Quays Sexual Health Clinic
- ChildLine (www.childline.org.uk)
- No Limits (www.nolimits.org.uk/goto/alcohol.html)
- It's Your Choice (www.connexions-direct.com/itsyourchoice/)
- Samaritans (www.samaritans.org)
- Rape Crisis (www.rapecrisis.org.uk)
- Youth Access (www.youthaccess.org.uk)
- The Rainbow Project (www.rainbow-project.org/dev/)

- If the home situation raises concerns, consider referral to Social Services. If you consider this to be urgent, contact the duty social worker. If not urgent, it can wait until the following day.
- Always remember that the young person can come to harm accidentally. If the young person's presentation placed them at significant risk (e.g. young female found unconscious in public place at risk of abduction), consider admission.
- Other concerning factors may include:
  - drinking alone
  - time of day
  - taken in conjunction with other drugs
  - intention (e.g. drinking socially with friends/or drinking to get drunk).

Parental supervision

If you decide not to admit the young person, ensure they are returning to a safe environment and responsible adult. If the environment concerns you, discuss with the on-call social worker. If appropriate, give telephone numbers of the drugs and alcohol team.

A patient with a Glasgow Coma Scale score of 15 may go home if:

- the patient is returning to a safe environment with a responsible adult;
- you do not believe the person or other people to be in danger and there are no major causes for concern as above.

Substance misuse

Most young peoeple that present with substance misuse do so as they are feeling unwell. Some may have underlying individual or family problems that need attention.

If, during your assessment, psychological concerns are raised:

- the younger the child, the greater your concern should be;
- if you believe the young person is in immediate danger (from themselves or others) consider admission;
- if the home situation raises concerns, consider referral to Social Services. If you consider this to be urgent, contact the duty social worker. If not urgent, it can wait until the following day;
- all young people presenting in this manner should be informed of voluntary services (e.g. No Limits (www.nolimits.org.uk/goto/alcohol.html), drugs and alcohol team);
- the young person should always be discharged to the care of a responsible adult.

Any concerns can always be discussed with the paediatric liaison team.

Self-harm (including cutting and self-injury)

- When presented with any form of self-harm, it is important to ask about suicidal ideas and intent.

- If the young person expresses suicidal intent, admit.
- The younger the child, the lower the threshold for admission should be.
- If you are unsure, discuss with the psychiatry team (or paediatric liaison team either via the relevant extension, or via the switchboard if out of hours/weekend/Bank Holiday).

If not admitted

- if not previously known, inform GP;
- all young people presenting in this manner should be informed of voluntary counselling services (Box V.i);
- assess degree of parental supervision.

If you decide not to admit, ensure the young person is returning to a safe environment and responsible adult. If the environment concerns you, discuss with the on-call social worker.

Example 2: Whittington Hospital, London

Criterion for use

For use by all staff dealing with patients in the emergency department up to their 18th birthday who have harmed themselves deliberately[2] by overdose or other means.

All must be referred directly to paediatrics for admission.

Emergency department staff

- Assess need for emergency treatment.
  - Paracetamol poisoning: please see Whittington Hospital NHS Trust guideline *Medical Management of Paracetamol Overdose*.
- Contact on-call senior house officer/middle-grade paediatrician.
  - In all cases a responsible adult must be contacted to attend the emergency department immediately and must remain with the patient until they have been admitted.
  - There are no grounds for concealing the fact of self-harm from the person with parental responsibility for any patient under 18.
  - Discharge direct from the emergency department is not acceptable practice.
  - If there is evidence of acute danger or serious mental illness refer to psychiatric management of under 18s.

---

2. This means that the person wanted to harm themselves, even if the dose or harm is minimal.

- Ascertain with paediatric ward staff what further assessment is necessary before accepting admission to ward. Is a telephone call describing the patient sufficient or should a nurse or doctor examine the patient in the emergency department?
- Please see Whittington Hospital NHS Trust guideline *Psychiatric Management of Under 18s in the Emergency Department*.

Paediatric medical and nursing staff

- Admit young person.
- Take detailed history.
  - Record accurately all significant names, addresses and telephone numbers including those of relevant professionals who have been involved with the patient or their family.
- Assess intent to self-harm.
  - Deliberate self-harm is self-inflicted injury and/or ingestion of substances with intent to self-harm or to die by suicide. This may include alcohol intoxication but only if the alcohol was consumed with an intent to self-harm. 'Cutting' is a serious symptom of despair and shame, even when the risk of suicide may be low.
  - The judgement as to whether the harm is accidental or deliberate is a clinical one to be made by paediatric staff. Accidental poisoning in younger children is obviously different, but some adolescents who have drunk too much alcohol may be desperate or even suicidal. Get a story and a background social history.
  - The dosage or method is less significant than the intent.
- Refer to child and family social work department.
  - The child and family social work department as lead practitioners will, accompanied by ward staff where possible, carry out risk assessment and initiate casework in liaison with child and adolescent psychiatry.
- Out of hours, admit in the usual way and wait for social work risk assessment the following morning.
  - If case cannot wait (too urgent or long weekend holiday), consult paediatric specialist registrar or on-call consultant and if then indicated contact duty[3] specialist registrar in child and adolescent psychiatry on call (via switchbhoard).

Guidelines for psychosocial risk assessment by doctors and nurses

This is NOT a protocol, i.e. don't just tick boxes, be curious about the self-harm and its personal and social context.

---

3. These specialist registrars are non-resident second on-call for three acute hospitals at the same time, to be called only after consultation with paediatric specialist registrars or consultants.

- What method did you use?
- If tablets were taken, were they yours or is there someone close to you who is ill or taking medication, or who has tried to harm themselves?
- Have you been ill or been given medication?
- Do you drink or use drugs?
- Did you plan to kill yourself?
- If so, for how long have you been thinking about it?
- How were you found; did you expect to be found?
- Did you regret what you did?
- What did you wish would happen?
- Have you made any previous attempts to harm yourself?
- Were the previous attempts more or less dangerous than this one?
- Did you leave a note? (Ask patient to show it to you or to repeat what it said.)
- Do you think a lot about death?
- Could you be mistaken (i.e. concealing the facts) about the time or quantity of overdose?
- What do you wish could happen now?

- You can ask the patient to score themselves on a scale of 0–10 of suicidal risk (almost everyone can respond quickly to this).
- It is safer to assume there was a wish to die, however transient, than to miss it. You can speak openly with the patient about suicidal thoughts. There is no risk of putting the idea into their head.
- Danger signals that increase the risk of suicide are:
  - hopelessness about the future
  - hostility
  - negative self-concept (i.e. the patient thinks they are a useless no-good person)
  - isolation.

Assessment of the patient's social network

- With whom do you live?
- Who and where are your parents and grandparents? (If dead ask for cause of death.)
- Use this data to make a three-generational family tree.
- Who are your closest friends/associates?
- Who are the most important people in your life?
- Is there anyone close to you that you are worried about?
- Besides parents or step-parents, do you have adult friends, a teacher/tutor, religious minister, young offenders worker, counsellor, social worker, psychiatrist, probation officer or other person whom you trust or who might be able to help? Have you seen such a person recently?

- Who is most likely to be able to help and why?
- What contact do you have with your GP?
- Has anyone close to you recently left, died or become ill?

Look out for recent exits (separation, leaving home, death) or entrances (new baby, new partner, other relative or friend) in the family or social network.

Sources of advice, information and contact

- Paediatric consultant attending or on call (via switchboard).
- Children and families social work team, Whittington Hospital.
- Consultant child and adolescent psychiatrists at Whittington Hospital (contact via switchboard). These are part-time staff who between them provide 0.6 whole time equivalents per week and backup on-call for duty specialist regisistrar out of hours.

Appendix VI
Emergency department mental health risk assessment tool

Diana Hulbert

Factors to be considered prior to initial assessment

- Has a physical cause been ruled out?
- Has drug and/or alcohol intoxication been ruled out?
- Is the patient well enough to be assessed?
- Is the patient known to the emergency department (check and use care plan if one exists)?
- Manage violence and aggression as per the emergency department policy

Following initial assessment (see below) screening for suicide risk is carried out. The patient is then put into a risk category depending on the answer given: red=high risk, orange=medium risk, and green=low risk.

Question	Yes	No
Background history/general observations		
_Is there an immediate risk of harm to self or others?	Red	Green
Is the patient aggressive and/or threatening?	Orange	Green
Is it likely that the patient will abscond?	Orange	Green
Is there a history of violence?	Orange	Green
Is there a history of self-harm?	Orange	Green
Is there a history of mental health problems?	Orange	Green
Appearance and behaviour		
Is the patient in obvious distress/markedly anxious/highly aroused?	Orange	Green
Is the patient behaving inappropriately?	Orange	Green
Is the patient quiet and withdrawn?	Orange	Green
Is the patient inattentive and uncooperative?	Orange	Green

Question	Yes	No
Issues explored through brief questioning		
Why is the patient presenting now/any triggers/recent events?		
What is the patient's level of social support?		
Are there major housing/accommodation issues?	Orange	Green
Does the patient appear to be experiencing delusions/hallucinations?	Red	Green
Does the patient feel controlled or influenced by external forces?	Red	Green

Index

Compiled by Caroline Sheard